MW01519087

Leona Choy

Leona Choy

HOSPITAL GOWNS

Don't HAVE POCKETS!

Why Me?
What now?

God will show us!

Published by
P.O. Box

Translated by Gail W.
Produced by Michael Th

Library of Congress

Troy, Leona
    Hospital Gowns

ISBN 1-889283-04
        1. Non-Fiction
            includes

Published in the United States

About the Author

Born of Czech parents in Iowa and a graduate of Wheaton College, Illinois, Leona Choy served with her late husband, Ted, in mission, church and educational work in Hong Kong, Singapore, China and the United States. Co-founder of *Ambassadors For Christ, Inc.*, a campus ministry for Chinese university students and scholars, her quarter century of work was administrative and editorial.

Fourteen trips to the People's Republic of China as guide/escort and English teaching consultant enriched her research and experiences for writing. As President of *WTRM-FM (Southern Light Gospel Music Network)* in the Shenandoah Valley of Virginia, Leona produced a daily radio program for five years.

Author, editor or collaborator of over 25 published books and 12 foreign language editions, her articles have appeared in over 70 different periodicals. Leona's poems have been published in scores of magazines and read over her daily radio programs, *Intensive Care,* and *Living It Up* on *WTRM.*

She is managing editor of *Golden Morning Publishing* in Winchester, Virginia, where she makes her home. Four grown sons and seven grandchildren keep her busy when she isn't writing or traveling.

Contents

About the Author
Dedication
Contents
Foreword

Part One
Pre-Op: Struggling

1. In the Admitting Room   /2
2. Jumping Over Hurdles   /9
3. Deserve It or Not?   /27
4. No Answer   /41
5. Am I Finished?   /60
6. No Wheeling Or Dealing   /76

Part Two
This is IT!: Submerged

7. Are We Having Fun Yet?   /98

Part Three
Post-Op:Emerging

8. Working My Way Through Spiritual College   /123
9. Dancing In Bed   /147

Part Four
Recovery and Reentry

10. Is There Life After Hospital?   /174
11. Downsittings and Uprisings   /196
12. Oil In My Water   /216
13. Bench Warming Lessons   /240
14. Trying to Add Cubits   /270

Endnotes   /293
Reading Resources   /295

The Back of the Book
Don't miss exploring this rich mine of valuable resources!

Life After Life   /297
Bible Promises About the Future   /301
Under the Master's Command   /303
Take time Out   /306
Just In Case   /311
Leona's Books   /314

Dedication

To God
whose I am and
who got me into this "on purpose"

To Dr. Jack Curtis, God's man
who wielded a skillful scalpel
to give me some bonus years to serve God

To my "cheer leader" Christian friends
across the world who prayed me through
and held me up when I was flying low

To my new reader friends
who work through this learning journey
with me and with God

To Edith, my good friend and buddy
in whom Christ dwells
on whom I tried out all the chapters
when she was jumping over surgical hurdles

To Gail, my gifted artist friend
creator of "GG the Bunny" drawings
who could fill hospital gown pockets
with her own illness-journey experiences
if they had pockets.

How blessed is he who considers the helpless; the Lord will deliver him in a day of trouble. The Lord will protect him, and keep him alive. . . .The Lord will sustain him upon his sickbed; in his illness, Thou dost restore him to health. As for me, I said, "O Lord, be gracious to me. . . .Blessed be the Lord. . . .Amen and amen."
(Selections from Psalm 41)

Foreword

My friend and soul mate for all but the first 16 years of my life, Leona Choy has validated her deep walk with the Lord and devotion to Him in yet another of her books, *Hospital Gowns.*

Having spent some of our teen years in the same Iowa town and nurtured in the same church, we went on to become classmates at Wheaton College. Our ways parted when we both married and served the Lord on our respective mission fields during most of our mid-years. But our close friendship was never interrupted and resumed even more intimately in our latter years.

Leona's personal friendship and her books have been a source of genuine enrichment in my own life. I cannot forget that she walked with me by prayer, phone and letters of encouragement during my surgical ordeal. This book is not platitudes but a "traveled through" and "prayed through" journey that is sure to impart hope, peace and courage so desperately needed as most of us eventually face some illness and accompanying surgical attention. She has bared her soul with utmost candor as to fears, hopes, doubts and assurances before, during and after her life-threatening cancer surgery. Readers cannot help identifying with her in every step and thus gaining help for their own experience.

Leona enriches the book by drawing upon many resources from the experiences and writings of others to share with us in this book. The BACK OF THE BOOK is packed with practical information that should not be missed.

Typical of the author, she didn't miss a beat or waste an experience. Her desire, as always, was to maximize the opportunity for God's kingdom and His people whom He calls upon to struggle through physical illness. *Hospital Gowns* reveals Leona's sensitive spirit as she interprets the deeper things of God to the needy and hungry soul facing some physical distress. There is an unveiling of Christ's love and presence you will be pleased to experience.

The "GG Bunny" drawings by Gail Waeber that introduce each chapter are delightful and meaningful. They help to lighten and balance the serious matters to which we are giving our attention. This is a "must" book you will want to recommend to any fellow pilgrim facing a hospital adventure or recovering.

Edith Lautz
Carol Stream, Illinois

Part 1

Pre-Op: Struggling

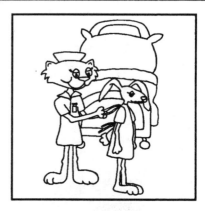

Chapter 1

In the Admitting Room

Wait a minute . . . who *wants* a hospital adventure?

I don't, and I believe you don't either. Illnesses, accidents and surgeries may happen to *other people,* but I never expect them to happen to me. I always keep the idea of illness at arm's length. I drive past hospitals thankful that I'm not lying in one of the antiseptic rooms.

However, most of us don't live out our lives without a hospital experience of some sort. Few reach Medicare age without entering the hospital as an outpatient or inpatient for some -oscopy, biopsy, x-ray, blood profile or other diagnostic "goodies." From then on the likelihood of an illness and hospitalization increases. It comes with the package of our mortal life on planet Earth.

Like it or not, some kind of illness or hospital adventure probably waits around the corner for you or your significant others before long. Let's face it—some friend or family member will suffer an illness or be involved in an accident. We are not being negative or asking for trouble; such happenings just occur as part of life.

Cheer up! Hospitals are ideal places not only for bodily repair jobs but excellent classrooms for soul-searching and life evaluation.

My hospital adventure caught me by surprise.

Other than a tonsillectomy at age 13 and four maternity experiences I steered clear of the admitting room. Suddenly I found myself working through my first and unexpected life-threatening journey. I share with you my fears and tears, trauma and drama, questions and apprehensions, yearnings and learnings, doubts and joyful shouts as I searched for meaning in the "friendly fire" into which I was catapulted.

You may be ahead of me in the school of illness, a graduate student in pain from the hallowed halls of hospitals. Perhaps you are a repeater in the emergency room. You may have wrestled through such emotions and found the answers to your questions long ago. I wish you had walked with me through my inner trauma so I could have benefitted from your counsel.

Perhaps you are a first-timer like I was. Or you may want to give this book to someone headed for the hospital or persons struggling through a recovery period but still working through some "whys."

We are here on purpose

No matter how this book came into your hands, I believe God meant it for some purpose. The problems you face and feelings you experience may not be the same as mine, but I invite you to walk with me through the illness tunnel. Your physical distress may not lead to hospitalization. Never mind. The principles are the same. Let's face our struggles together and hold hands for support. An important learning experience lies ahead of us.

This is not a "let me tell you about my operation" book. In fact, you don't even have to go into surgery with me. Feel free to skip that chapter. Nor is this the last word on how to encounter and make our way through an illness. Some of the questions which bombard us may have no immediate answers. Perhaps my thoughts can be catalysts to help you explore ways of coping with physical distress. God tutors us personally as we listen to Him.

The thoughts in this book were written as I worked through my own experience. I invite you to walk in my hospital slippers with me. Consider this an interactive book. Go ahead and make notes in the margins. Use a highlighter to emphasize thoughts and feelings with which you identify. Scribble *Yes!* where you agree, *No!* where you don't, or *?* where you are still struggling or uncertain. Keep your Bible handy. I have laced the text with Scripture references that are relevant to our situation, either quoted or for you to look up and internalize.

You may use the "Personal Workout" questions at the end of each chapter to work through privately. You don't have to show your answers to anyone. A study group may also use the questions as discussion starters.

Don't leave home without it!

I wrote from the viewpoint of my Christian faith and with the assurance that my loving Heavenly Father planned my hospital adventure "on purpose." It wasn't a random happening. Although it appeared negative and harmful, God intended it for my spiritual growth and for His glory. I certainly didn't ask for it or thought I needed it; apparently the Lord knew I did.

Without personal faith in Jesus Christ I would be afraid to go through any illness or march into any hospital adventure. In fact, to live day by day without being "in Christ" is to take unnecessary, eternal risks. A life without faith in God is hazardous to the health of both your soul and body.

If *you* don't yet enjoy the assurance of a personal faith in Jesus Christ, *please,* before you read further, turn to the brief last section in *The Back of the Book* titled "Life After Life." That's the place to *start!* Don't leave home for the hospital or anywhere else without it— without God. We don't need to walk through illness alone. God is with us on the journey! In fact, He has the steering wheel in His sovereign hands.

What's this about pockets?

The title of this book may have made you curious. When we enter the hospital and shed our street clothes, we discover that most of the gowns we wear *don't have pockets.* Apparently we don't need any. A sheet of instructions given before admission spells out: "Leave your valuables at home. This includes money, watch, credit cards, jewelry and contact lenses." When I slip into my without-pockets hospital gown, it's obvious that I can't bring my personal, educational or professional reputation with me. No one cares about my achievements and expertise. I'm literally stripped to bare essentials. My "designer gown" is the ultimate leveler of humanity!

When I lie on the operating table, I'm a generic, "equal opportunity" patient. What the surgical team does for me and to me doesn't depend on who I am, what I've done or what I still hope to do. My identity doesn't matter to them beyond checking (I hope!) my plastic I.D. bracelet to see if I'm the right body to receive the scheduled operation.

Why is this piece of clothing called a "gown?" We usually think of gowns as fashionable attire for formal occasions. Surgery is about as informal as you can get!

Gowns in doctors' examination rooms are usually made of paper and are disposable. They remind me that all things in life are temporary. My physical distress, too, will pass. Some gowns are like large vests with no sleeves. Sometimes the nurse tells me to put the unmanageable thing on with the opening at the back, sometimes at the front, depending on what the doctor wants to peer at or poke. Some are street-length paper gowns without fasteners. *Never with pockets.*

Gowns they issue to us in the hospital are hardly more fashionable than exam room gowns, although made of cloth and more durable. Sometimes they are white, drab green or blue. Some have a tiny logo of the admitting hospital in an overall design. Hospital gowns apparently start out with strings to tie, but more often than not at least one string is missing. (Who is being treated so roughly?) In the shortie gowns I'm exposed and drafty on my backside.

I confess that during my periodic x-rays as an outpatient during recovery years I wore a gown or two that *did* have pockets. Never mind . . . they weren't *hospital gowns.* A friend did tell me that her special issue hospital gown had a pocket right in front center for carrying a heart monitor. I'll concede that exception, but I won't change my book title!

Ready, set, GO!

The nurse instructed me to stuff my street clothes and shoes into what looked like a white garbage bag provided by the hospital. I wondered, *Will I ever wear my clothes again?*

"Ready?" she asked cheerfully from outside the curtain.

I took a deep breath, pulled aside the curtain and emerged from my preparatory cubicle for better or worse. I stood unsteady in my terry cloth slippers with rubber soles. *No way am I ready for what is coming!*

Likewise, I will stand before God, my Creator and Judge, when I arrive in His presence on that Final Reckoning Day. I blink. *What if it is today?* For that event I should be ready.

My gown on That Day will also be provided. That garment *won't have pockets either.* No place for valuables, credentials, bank books, business cards or property deeds. No place for credit reports or references documenting my character, accomplishments or proficiency. I'll leave everything behind. "Just as I am without one plea but that Thy blood was shed for me, O Lamb of God, I come, I come."

I'll either be clothed in the righteousness of Jesus Christ, my Redeemer, or I'll be spiritually naked, without covering. My garment won't be earned or deserved, and I can't buy it at the door. It is made of clean, white linen, and I have to reserve it in advance.

The garment God gives to those who belong to Him has a "Whosoever" designer label, and one size fits all. ◆

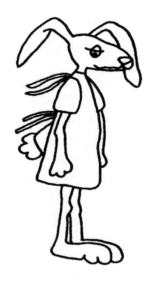

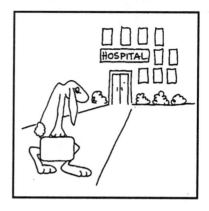

Chapter 2

Jumping Over Hurdles

Let's rewind the video tape to explore some struggles we may have *before* we arrive in the hospital admitting room.

My illness seemed like a race track of hurdles. I didn't sign up to enter this race, didn't think I qualified or had time to train for it. How could I jump those hurdles? Were they road blocks meant to stop me? Were they detours? Each hurdle looked as high as a mountain. I had to jump over each without missing any. The hurdles were my questions:

- Who caused my illness, God or Satan?
- What did I do to deserve this?
- Can God heal me? Will He?

- Should I exercise faith and refuse to accept my illness?
- Could my life be over?
- Is this a test from God?
- What's the worst case scenario?
- For what purpose might God bring this into my life?
- Is my illness a friend or an enemy?
- Why does God seem so far away?
- What if I have no way out but to go through this?

I thought I was following God's leading for my life, but this illness stopped me short. I had different plans. I was ready to leave for an overseas ministry trip. I had arranged my itinerary, bought my plane ticket and packed my suitcases. How could a routine, annual physical checkup suddenly change all that?

Of course I know that the Christian life isn't a deep pile red carpet to heaven or a magic carpet on which I float over the bumps of life. The Bible tells me that when difficulties test my faith, I shouldn't be surprised. *But I am!*

I know God sometimes speaks through adversities to His children. If He brought this illness to signal a detour, I'd better take it. If it's a road block, I'd better pay attention. If a test, I should do my best to get a passing grade. I shouldn't panic. *But I do.* Since I sincerely seek God's will, surely He will let me know why He brought me to face this monstrous mountain. He will take me over all the hurdles that lead to it.

Time is not on my side. Decisions come thick and fast. I must leap the hurdles quickly one after the other. I need God's light on the track ahead because I can't run in the darkness of my own understanding. The Bible instructs me:

> Trust in the Lord with all your heart, and do not lean on your own understanding. In all your ways acknowledge Him, and He will make your paths straight. (Proverbs 3:5,6)

> For Thou dost light my lamp; the Lord my God illumines my darkness. For by Thee I can run upon a troop; and by my God I can leap over a wall. (Psalm 18:28,29)

I must quickly internalize the adrenalin of God's promises. Since God says His light is shining on the darkness of my questions, I must start leaping the hurdles *now.*

Are you mad at me, God?

In a TV commercial for upgrading the contents of children's brown bag lunches, a disappointed little boy examined the lunch his mother packed for him. He didn't like what he found. He asked, "Are you mad at me, Mommy?"

I take this illness personally. I can't help it. I feel as if I'm getting something distasteful. I am God's child, but I don't like what my Heavenly Father is giving me for lunch.

Since I'm a Christian, I believe God is involved in my life. So He must have designed this trial for me. It is also true that much suffering comes as a result of living in a flawed world among spiritually fallen people. Moreover, rebellious spirit beings are active on planet Earth.

Some problems we even bring on ourselves.

Why do we accuse God and get mad at Him at the first hint of trouble? We overlook all other causes and lay the blame directly on His doorstep. When things go well, God may be the last one to whom we give credit.

God doesn't do anything to His children from anger. I know that. If I find something in my life-lunch that doesn't suit my taste, I am sure He put it there for my spiritual nourishment and my good. I wouldn't be spiritually healthy if He packed it daily with nothing but sweets. I wouldn't appreciate the sweets if they didn't contrast with some bitters of life.

Honest with God

Everything hinges on my positive response to my calamitous situation, but my halo is askew. I don't always have bright, shiny, positive responses. Not even most of the time.

Dark, negative thoughts lurk in the shadowy corners of my mind, and I can't seem to muster up the strength to take the broom of faith and sweep them out.

Those negative thoughts are not meek and quiet creatures. To my embarrassment, they are loud and brash. They even yell at God. But I know God will not give up on me even when pain squeezes negative complaints from me toward Him.

I believe God wants me to express honest thoughts and feelings to Him rather than hide behind pious expressions that I speak hypocritically. It doesn't matter what people expect or what I expect of myself, I need to be honest with God. Stephen Brown suggests:

> If you are angry and hurt . . . tell God the truth. He might be the only Person in the world who can absorb everything you hand Him, understand why you do it, and still love you.
>
> Too often, when our ropes have broken, our prayers become spiritual nonsense. If we would stop talking nonsense for a moment, God would say to us, "Come off it! Tell me what you really think." Once we believers, who have had ropes break, understand that God can handle our honesty, the broken ropes don't seem as bad as they seemed before. [1]

I don't think God will send a bolt of lightning to zap me if I tell Him how I *really* feel. If I can't be honest with Him, I can't be honest with anyone. Besides, since He knows everything, even my thoughts, He already knows how I feel. I guess I vent my feelings to Him mostly for my benefit. So here it goes:

God, I'm hurt because You let this happen to me when I thought I was walking in Your ways.

I'm confused because You didn't let me know sooner that You were going to set aside my plans. Why did You let me go to the last minute? I did consult You about my plans.

I'm disappointed because I don't think I deserve to go through this affliction.

I'm puzzled because I don't know what You are after in my life.

I'm jealous of others who disregard You yet they

aren't suffering or ill.

I feel that You abandoned me because You are silent when I ask You questions. Now is the time I most need to hear from You!

I don't feel spiritual. I feel like pouting and crying. If I told you otherwise, God, I'd be lying, and I don't think You'd like that.

Truly, I'm scared. Scared to death!

There—I've let it all hang out.

The air is clearer between us. I still don't hear any answers from You, nor do I see any handwriting on the wall, but I know in my heart of hearts that You do love me. The universe doesn't really revolve around me . . . You are the center and Your big sovereign plan is in action.

How does God work things out?

I'm trying to figure out how You work, Lord: If I'm "good," doesn't it mean that I won't suffer or have reverses? No? You say that isn't the way it works? Those who are "bad" may not receive Your judgment in this life? Therefore, I shouldn't expect the "Santa Claus policy" to apply? That You won't necessarily reward me with good gifts if I'm on good behavior? Or withhold good gifts from me if I'm disobedient or willful? Apparently, not only super-spiritual people qualify to have their prayers answered.

What about bad things happening to godly people? And good things happening to people who enjoy being bad, flout Your laws, abuse their bodies and laugh in Your face? Many of them are healthy and seem to get away with their evil deeds. (Psalm 73) Don't You reward us now, in this life, for sincerely following You?

I guess the key word is "now."

You created a perfect planet, and it was Your decision to give free will to the human beings You created. Unfortunately, man exercised his free will and disobeyed You. Suffering and death resulted, and the natural world was cursed. One day You will restore it to its pristine perfection. *But not yet.* You will abolish suffering. *But not yet.* You will judge all sin. *But not yet.* You will reward obedience. *But not yet.* (2 Peter 2:4-9) Things will be evened up and fairness will reign. *But not yet.*

For now, we face inequities and injustices. (2 Peter 3:9) When Jesus comes again and sets up His kingdom on earth as He promised, You will straighten everything out, right?

That comforts me! Yes, God, I'm beginning to understand Your ways a little better.

I want it all explained—*now*

If I could understand the reasons for my situation—the current reasons, the long-range ones, the ultimate reasons—I think I could more easily go through this trial.

Perhaps. Maybe not. Well, *probably* not.

If God showed me a completed, full-color and stereo "This is your life!" documentary, and I clearly knew where I'm headed and why, what would I do? If He showed me that my earthly road ahead is treacherous, I would probably dig in my heels and refuse to go on. If God lifted the veil and let me see that my future is packed with pleasure, I would be too impatient for it all to work out.

God doesn't owe me any explanation. I don't need to know, nor should I expect to understand right now where this unhappy segment I'm going through fits into His plan. God's vantage point is eternal. What is happening to me right now is already past in His eternal view. I should trust God with what I don't see because of my human limitations.

God is not obligated to tell me what His purposes are or what part in them I should play. It pleases Him when I, as His created one, show faith and confidence in His ultimate plan. I can see only this day, this moment. It is enough for me to know that God is in control of everything.

Lord, give me the patience to trust You and hang on even if I can't find meaning in what I am going through. I don't want to mouth syrupy spiritual platitudes that haven't been worked out in the nitty-gritty of my life. Help me be real.

"Who done it?"

Before I can deal with my situation, I wrestle with the question of where it came from. Not necessarily my immediate illness or affliction, but "first cause," the source, the origin. I want to know who is behind the curtain.

Even Christians don't agree about first cause. Some are convinced that all illness, pain, suffering and affliction must come from the devil. That we should drive our illness away because it is an evil thing. We should take authority over it, not accept it, declare that it isn't there, count it as already gone. They believe nothing bad could possibly come from a good God. Some of Job's self-styled counselors insisted that his calamities came because of his personal sin, that he was suffering God's judgment and punishment.

Scripture is my only reliable source, and the decision of the Judge (God) is final. I am qualified to claim the promise in Romans 8:28 because I belong to the Lord. "We know that God causes all things to work together for good to those who love God, to those who are called according to His purpose." I can be sure that whatever I'm going through must be *God-ordained.* It originated with Him, or He allowed it to happen, planned it for His good and for my good.

Obviously, "all things" means everything. The good and pleasant things, certainly, but also afflictions, sicknesses, distresses, natural catastrophes and accidents. The apostle Paul gave several lists of such things. "All" must include my particular situation.

But how can God be in control when life seems so out of control? How can He be working things together for His glory and our ultimate good? Warren Wiersbe in his book *Why Us?* states it well:

> God proves His sovereignty not by intervening constantly and preventing these events but by ruling and overruling them so that even tragedies end up accomplishing His ultimate purposes.

So then, *"who done it?"* I simply don't know. I don't need to know, nor do I need to run interference for God or defend His integrity. I don't pretend to fully understand the reasons for the suffering that either I or others may experience. What God wants to accomplish in one person may be entirely different from His working in the life of another.

It follows that I don't dare to say God must heal a particular person on a given occasion because I don't know what He is working out in that person's life. I might hinder God's will if I demand healing for him or for myself.

Will I accept the package?

My problem is like a package delivered to my door. It is something I don't want and haven't ordered. As God's child, do I have the option of pushing it away, if I see that the return address is *His?*

There seems to be something inherently unchristian to refuse to accept an illness or some negative circumstance *because it can't possibly come from the God of love.* Do we dare say, "Return to sender"? Only if we are absolutely certain that *God* has not sent it or allowed it in our lives for His sovereign purpose could we even consider rejecting it. But can any of us be *that* certain with our finite minds? We can't second-guess God. His ways remain a mystery beyond our comprehension. (Isaiah 55:8,9) Since God sends or allows *everything* in the life of a Christian, is there ever a time when we should say *no* and refuse anything?

I would be spiritually presumptuous if I insist on rejecting or resisting what a loving and just God offers me. As Job said, "Shall we accept good at the hand of God and not evil?" Moreover, it won't work. I can't prevail against Him. He will have His way.

Making it personal, if I resist God's dealings with

me through this present affliction, I may resist God Himself. I push aside His hand of love. I rebel against Him and am disobedient. If I automatically declare that every affliction comes straight from the devil, I might attribute God's work in me to a Satanic source. A risky spiritual premise!

Charles Stanley counsels:

> The way you respond when God is behind [adversity] and the way you respond when Satan is behind it is *identical.* This may come as a surprise. But think about it. Most of the time you really do not know who is behind it. *And it really does not matter.* What is important is your response. If God is behind it, He is going to use it for your good. If Satan is behind it, you know he works under God's supervision. God uses even Satan's schemes to accomplish His will. You are not pressed to discover the source, but *you are expected to respond correctly.* . . . As long as God is accomplishing His purpose through the adversity in your life, you can receive it as if it were from Him. [2]

How much better to open my hand and accept what God sends, offer my hand to Him and move on to walk through the learning experience He lovingly planned for me. If God chooses to change the circumstances, it will be good. If He does not, it will also be good.

Jesus agonized in prayer asking to be spared from "the cup" of suffering ahead . . . if it were His Father's will. Paul repeatedly pleaded for God to remove his "thorn in the flesh." In both cases, cup and thorn, it was for God's glory and for the eternal benefit of mankind that God did not grant those requests.

Yes, Lord, yes!

At the beginning of my journey into this surgical adventure I need to settle the matter of acceptance. Facing the unknown, I want to shake my head *no* to whatever is coming instead of nodding *yes*. The Lord is going to do His loving, though painful, spiritual surgery on me anyway. It will be much easier on me if I joyfully sign an unconditional consent form and give it to Him. Then my heels won't get sore from digging in because He won't have to drag me along kicking and screaming.

The words of a gospel song come to mind:

> *Yes, Lord, Yes!* to Your will and to Your way.
> *Yes, Lord, Yes!* I will trust You and obey.
> When Your Spirit speaks to me,
> with my whole heart I'll agree,
> and my answer will be Yes, Lord, Yes!

My positive outlook is not a cure-all. It won't change facts, but it does change me. That is not like the half-truth, "If you say it, you have it." I can't treat the God of the universe like a genie in a bottle who grants me three wishes whenever I rub Him the right way. I don't understand how it works, but my attitude of submission to God's Plan "A" for me infuses a kind of healing, spiritual medication into my mind and body. Medical science agrees that attitude plays a major part in healing and recovery. A negative attitude puts me on a sled and gives me a fast push downhill.

The disciple Peter learned the hard way. Devoted but impulsive, he often blurted out the first thing that popped into his head. When Jesus informed His disciples that He had to go to Jerusalem to suffer and die, Peter jumped right in with a protest, "No, Lord, no!" Jesus actually addressed the devil in Peter by saying, "Get behind me, Satan!" If I maintain a negative, denial attitude, I act as if I know more than God. How can I say *no* and *Lord* in the same breath? One cancels the other.

Like Job in the Bible record, I don't know what's going on behind the curtain in the unseen spiritual realm. But I believe that the *source* of an illness, an accident or what seems to be an adversity, is not as important as *my attitude or response toward God*.

Triumphing with the Lord through an illness seems a better spiritual stance than fighting it, denying it or insisting that He blow it away. Cooperating with Him and with medical science in the steps of the healing process expresses *Yes, Lord, yes.* I have the joyful opportunity to please the Lord by listening to Him when He's trying to tell me what He wants to do with me, in me, through me in this illness.

My Heavenly Father knows that I'm responding to Him and not to Satan. Satan may eavesdrop if he can because then he will be sure I'm not accepting *his* infernal work.

The posture most pleasing to the Lord is for me to accept His will without reservation. Acceptance is different from resignation or fatalism. It is positive affirmation. Resignation is negatively passive. It gives up and quits. Acceptance moves on.

No matter what it may say on the outside of the wrapper of whatever happens to me, it's *always* a "Hallelujah package" sent from God.

If I find out that there's no way but through, and that God is leading me in His love and for His purpose down this path of affliction, I'm going to receive it and squeeze every ounce of good from the experience. That brings my present distress into a new dimension!

Although they may wheel me on a gurney under anesthesia *from* the O.R., I can march *into* the experience of surgery, if that becomes necessary, by accepting my God-given assignment. If God says, "Take it from Me," I'll receive it.

That doesn't mean I'm brave. Actually, I'm afraid. "Not that we are adequate in ourselves to consider anything as coming from ourselves, but our adequacy is from God" (2 Corinthians 3:5). No doubt about it, God will have to carry me on the wings of *His* courage, *His* strength and *His* adequacy. "But thanks be to God, who gives us the victory in our Lord Jesus Christ" (1 Corinthians 15:57).

A plastic bubble?

Why do I think it's unusual to suffer an illness when I've tried to be God's obedient child? Do I assume that God should shield me from all the difficulties other people face?

I've lived long enough to understand that God doesn't enclose His children inside a big protective plastic bubble. Jesus prayed, "I do not ask Thee to take them out of the world, but to keep them from the evil one" (John 17:15).

As part of humanity, I'm subject to whatever happens on planet Earth. I live in a fallen world among fallen, unregenerate men and women and in a flawed natural environment. I can't expect to escape the adversities, afflictions, misfortunes and calamities common to mankind. I'm still exposed to illnesses that may be contagious. I can be involved in an accident. My body goes through the normal aging process and the eventual deterioration and dysfunction of organs. I will experience physical death when God's time comes to take me Home. If natural disasters like floods, tornados or earthquakes occur, I may not escape injury just because I'm a Christian. I can't avoid breathing some polluted air, eating some food with harmful chemical additives or grown with lethal pesticides.

The hedge that the Bible says God put around His servant Job was invisible but nonetheless real. God didn't give Satan permission to step beyond His spiritual protection. Job's soul was out-of-bounds to Satan's power or interference. In John 10:10, Jesus spoke of the devil as a thief who comes only to steal, kill and destroy. Jesus, on the other hand, came to give us life abundantly.

The devil can't steal from me unless I let him. God won't let him. The devil can't destroy that which is truly valuable to me because I've already stored it in God's Federal Reserve Bank in heaven. Satan has no access code to that walk-in bank vault.

God has planted a spiritual hedge around His redeemed sons and daughters. Jesus said, "Don't be afraid of those who can kill only your bodies but can't touch your souls! Fear only God who can destroy both soul and body in hell" (Matthew 10:28TLB).

Satan couldn't touch Job's soul no matter what happened to his body, his family or possessions. Since I belong to the Lord, whatever happens to me in this life occurs *outside* the hedge that God has put around my soul. Nothing can harm my eternal welfare.

Jesus described two houses, symbolically two lives, one built on sand, the other on a rock. The same wind and rain and floods came upon both houses, but the result was different because of the foundation. Our foundation is the Rock of Ages—God.

The bubble in which I'm safe is God's love and care and plan. Nothing can reach me there unless God allows it for His perfect purpose. Therefore, I'm not to wonder, not to worry, only to trust God. His bubble will never self-destruct, and the devil's pin can't burst it. ◆

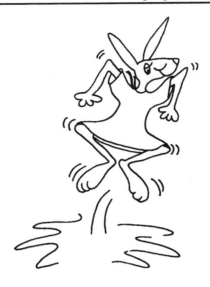

My Personal Workout

1. Do I assume that my illness comes from the devil? Why isn't that necessarily so?

2. How did suffering, evil and sickness come into God's perfect world? How might I suffer from the world's present flawed condition?

3. When will God straighten out all the injustices and inequities in the world?

4. Do I accept or reject my physical affliction? Why?

5. Is my predominant attitude toward God one of acceptance or resistance?

6. What changes might take place in my life if I stopped negative thinking?

7. Do I insist that God explain immediately the reasons for my illness?

8. Do I assume that God should protect me from the difficulties of life just because I'm a Christian?

9. How can I move forward to a deeper faith and trust in God?

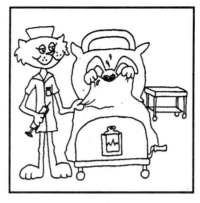

Chapter 3

Deserve It or Not?

If I had a daisy, I'd tear the petals off one by one: "Deserve it . . . deserve it *not* . . . deserve it . . . deserve it *not*. . . ." Deserve what? This catastrophe (as I look at it).

Is my physical trauma a punishment? If I abused my body by taking in improper substances or treated it carelessly, it might be a consequence of such abuse. Or it might be the result of something I did or failed to do, or which was done to me. In such cases, if I am God's child, it would still not be a *punishment*. I would simply have brought it on myself, and therefore I deserve it.

If I brought on my illness by my own actions, I don't want to ask for God's *justice*. I would get what I deserve. I want to ask for God's *mercy*. Spiritually, I already received God's mercy and forgiveness for my sins through trusting Christ. God's justice would have brought me His judgment and punishment, which I deserve.

But whether or not I receive God's mercy when my illness is the consequence of my wrongdoing or indulgences is up to His perfect will and plan. "I may get it . . . I may not . . . I may get it . . . I may not. . . ."

On the *other* hand, what if my illness is the result of accident, natural disaster, contagious disease, heredity or an environmental cause? All of us, Christians and unbelievers, are subject to nature's forces and human frailty. We must expect, accept and live through such things—or live with them, endure them, triumph over them and live in Christ's victory.

If *none* of these seem to be contributing factors to my illness, then what? I may question, *What did I do to deserve this?* Do I infer that I'm too good, too righteous, too obedient to the Lord to have anything "bad" happen to me?

My friends or family, perhaps not realizing that they reinforce my self-righteousness, rush in with "You're such a good person! Why should you have to suffer?" That doesn't foster a healthy attitude in me or a Christian one. I don't reflect the humility of a created one before my Creator.

Humility in the sense of modest submissiveness, gentle, patient yieldedness to God's dealings is more appropriate for me as His trusting child. This is not spineless submission, but confident belief in my sovereign God and a commitment to conform to His blueprint for my life.

Life is seldom fair. In fact, to use a crude term, sometimes life stinks!

I have a lot to think through and work out:

Is God really in charge? If He is, why does He seem so inconsistent when He allows one person to suffer and not another, heals this one and not that one? Why does He allow natural disasters to affect some and not others?

I believe the Bible teaches that Satan has power, though limited, to mess up God's perfect order at this stage of history. Satan tries to thwart God's plans, but God is in ultimate control even over Satan's continual infernal attempts at disorder.

I believe that God generously gave mankind freedom of choice. We can choose God's way or reject it to follow our own. Nevertheless, God knows what will happen. Sometimes He supernaturally intervenes on behalf of His people. Sometimes He doesn't.

Sometimes He allows us to be targets of evil people, bad genes, dangerous viruses or natural disasters without intervening. Hebrews chapter eleven lists some who escaped tragedies and experienced miracles. But a dreadful list follows of equally godly people who endured incredible sufferings. They were tortured, imprisoned, mocked, beaten, stoned, sawn in half, stabbed, ill-treated and stripped of everything for Jesus' sake. Such conditions continue across the world today.

God doesn't act on a whim or sometimes look the other way with indifference. He doesn't draw straws to see who should escape and who should suffer, who should get cancer at 45 and who should live a robust life to age 95.

Man's mistakes or deliberate acts of evil can affect other people and conditions on this planet, which in turn affect me. But of this I am sure—*God is good.* His dealings with me are for good and not evil. "'For I know the plans that I have for you,' declares the Lord, 'plans for welfare and not for calamity to give you a future and a hope'" (Jeremiah 19:11). Whatever good or evil comes into the life of one committed to follow God, even as part of the human condition, is not accidental. I have finite understanding. If I never discover the reason for my illness, I'll understand it when I leave my house (my mortal body) and arrive in God's house.

I believe God is involved in the minutia of human activity, incredible as that seems. Jesus stated that the very hairs of our head are numbered and He even knows when a sparrow falls. Therefore, I believe that my present circumstances aren't random happenings. If I could understand perfectly, I would be God, and I'm not.

The whole scenario may seem inconsistent and out-of-control to my way of thinking, but it is perfectly consistent from God's infinite viewpoint. The point is not that God *will be* sovereign some day, meanwhile evil forces and human actions mess up His plans. *Our God reigns now!* (Psalm 93:1) Everywhere! Always! Since I've voluntarily given Him my life, He reigns and He is sovereign *in my present trouble.*

This mortal life is not all there is! If it were, I'd feel short-changed and cheated. Life is so brief. We barely get started and gain a little experience when the final bell rings. Nor is human history all there is. I should look at my miniature infirmity (although it seems enormous to me) against the backdrop of eternity. Not easy, but that's the only way I can gain proper perspective and find the stability I need to endure even the worst that life may inflict. Our God stands above all human history and is weaving it into a beautiful tapestry that will ultimately glorify Him.

I believe, Lord. Help my lingering unbelief and increase my faith. I don't get anywhere when I destroy daisy petals to find out whether I deserve my situation. It's enough to believe that You know, care and have plans for me.

But why *me?*

Illness, surgery, accident—I ask myself, and I may ask others, *why me?* Eventually I knock on God's door and whine *why?* Other people are sympathetic and may also express *but why you?* The questions are always there. Answers are illusive, but let's pursue them further. *Why* questions can strangle me and take over my life. They may destroy my emotional balance and impede my potential recovery.

Dr. James Dobson gave an illustration from nature. He had a sturdy, ancient oak tree in his yard. A threatening, tenacious vine crept along a fence nearby. Before long, the vine headed for his tree, crept up the trunk and silently attacked it. Tough, green tentacles gripped the thick oak and imbedded themselves like claws in a hostile takeover.

Dr. Dobson didn't want to forcibly tear the vine off the healthy tree because much of the bark would come with it and leave the tree exposed. Besides, the vine would only seize hold elsewhere, and the battle would continue to rage.

His only recourse was to take big nippers and sever the vine at the root. The first day he saw no change in the vine. Then the leaves began to wither and lose color. Soon they became brown and brittle, and the fuzzy fingers loosened their grip. Dr. Dobson took a rake and easily pulled down the whole dry, messy mass and freed the oak to continue its vigorous life. The vine didn't give up permanently because the root remained underground, but he dealt with new sprouts more easily as they appeared.

If I keep wrestling with *why* this is happening to me, and allow the doubting questions to multiply and take over my thinking and grip my emotions, the vine of distrust and doubt in the sovereign goodness of God will choke me. My attitude will block my understanding of the higher ways of God. After all, I only comprehend a fraction of my diminutive personal world because I am a limited mortal. There will always be things I won't understand about God's plan for my life. Unanswered questions may plague me until the day I see His face.

I must simply believe that God is in control, knows what He is doing and that this seeming negative event is somehow for my good and His glory. I must let God be God without sniveling to Him about things I can't understand.

I should take an axe to my root of doubt and chop off the whimpering *whys* before they strangle my trust in God. The *whys* will wither and dry on the vine and then I can pull them away from me. Each time a green sprout of doubt peeks its head through the grass I must nip it off before it grips my faith trunk.

The vine might even be poison ivy! If I allow it to grow on me, not only will I suffer, but its doubts will spread infectiously to others whom my miserable life touches.

Why not?

There's another approach to questions with which I grapple. I can turn the big question "Why me?" into "Who better for it to happen to?"

As a loving Father, God provides me with unlimited resources at His disposal. So, who is better equipped for a calamity than the child of God?

The person who *doesn't* have an authentic relationship with God (because of his own choice) is really without adequate resources to meet inevitable troubles, trials and catastrophes. Random things without divine purpose *can* happen to him for which his *why* cries truly have *no answer.* Romans 8:28 *doesn't* apply to him. The Bible *doesn't* guarantee that God is meshing gears for good in the life of the not-trusting-God person.

For me as God's child, through no merit of my own, only by faith in Jesus, the seal upon my life is: "For we are His workmanship, created in Christ Jesus for good works, which God prepared beforehand, that we should walk in them" (Ephesians 2:10). God isn't going to shackle my feet through this so-called negative happening to hinder me from walking freely in His ways. My Lord is more likely to put liberating wings on my heels. Could the difficult experience I'm going through be a shiny new pair of heel wings releasing me to soar to heights I never experienced?

Why not me? If heel wings come with the package, I'll gladly accept it!

I already know there is *a purpose* in everything I go through. Nothing catches God by surprise. He brought the present illness into my life for His reasons, and they are always good. *Always!*

It's awesome to think of all the *supplements* God gives me over and above the medical facilities and physicians' skills available even to the patient who doesn't have a relationship with God.

♦ God gives me His presence, promises and provisions for my weakness. I have an "insider" person—the Person of the Holy Spirit—living in me as my Comforter, the One called alongside to help.

♦ God gives me His *joy* no matter how excruciating the circumstances.

♦ His *peace,* passing all human understanding, is mine to bring me through in triumph.

♦ I have an incredible *support system* in the fellowship of Christians called the church, the body of Christ, which will not let me down.

♦ I have *hope* in the wonderful eternity ahead of me whether by life or by death. Either way, I can't lose!

Whatever lies ahead of me, I don't need to get bent out of shape. In fact, God is working on my shape—He is conforming me to the image of Jesus Christ!

The ultimate "whatever"

Can God heal me? *Can* He deliver me? Does He *want* to? *Will* He? I need straight answers to those questions.

If I say He *can't,* He would not be God. He would be impotent and ineffective. He wouldn't be supernatural. Of course He *can!* He can do even what we consider impossible.

Does God *want* to heal me? Does He *want* to

deliver me? I am sure from the promises of His Word that God wants only good for His children and not evil. He wants what is best for my welfare and His glory.

Will God heal me? *Will* God deliver me? That is what I don't know because I can't see the Big Plan of God. I don't know whether an immediate supernatural healing or a surgery or my death at this time will be in *His* best interests and *mine* for time and eternity.

I'll take the position of Shadrach, Meshach and Abednego as recorded in Daniel chapter three. When faced with the prospect of being thrown into the furnace of blazing fire ending in sure death, they expressed their faith in God by declaring, "Our God whom we serve *is able to deliver us* from the furnace of blazing fire; and He will deliver us out of your hand, O king. *But even if He does not,* let it be known to you, O king, that we are not going to serve your gods or worship the golden image that you have set up" (vv. 17,18).

God *can.* But even if He *doesn't,* I'm going to trust Him. His deliverance may take a different direction.

Yes, I've asked God to intervene, to touch me, to heal me, to take away the abnormality I suffer. He is well able! I'm dealing with the Creator of the universe and the re-creator and restorer of anything. His *ability* is not in question.

To leave the outcome to Him means that whatever He decides I accept. He keeps the rest of the planet and universe in harmony, so He knows how my small event fits into it all. It's O.K. I won't stamp my feet to insist on a miraculous or instantaneous physical healing. For His best reasons God may have planned to lead me into the furnace and through the fire. If so, I'm sure He will appear there with me as He did with those courageous fellows in Babylon's oven.

The ultimate "whatever" is that I must leave the decision with Almighty God and declare obediently, "not my will be done but Thine." It wasn't easy for Jesus when He faced suffering. God didn't keep Him from it, although He could have. It's not easy for me, but it's a one-way street, and I can't turn back.

Asking for magic?

There's nothing I'd like better than a disappearing act—either misdiagnosis or to have my illness suddenly vanish. That would be my kind of miracle! God's kind of miracle may be different.

If it is magic we beg God for, we will be disillusioned. If it is meaning, purpose, strength, character, love and greatness we expect from Him in the midst of our difficulty, then He won't disappoint us. God may actually rescue us from going any further toward a hospital adventure. If He does, we can be certain it was best, and we can praise Him for it. Nevertheless, to rescue us or not is God's call, not ours. Praise should be our response in *either* case.

O.K., so I'm not looking for magic, but I know God can heal me instantly. He can do a disappearing act on my illness like He has done many times for many people, including me. Why doesn't He stretch out His hand to touch me with His healing power as I stretch my hands and spirit up to Him? "Yesterday, today, and forever He is the same" (Hebrews 13:8).

He is the same miracle-working God He always was. So why does He seem to be sitting on His hands *this time?*

John the Baptist, cast into prison and facing death, was in a life-threatening situation. Jesus surely cared about him and could have delivered him from impending death instantly. But He didn't. He could have commanded John's immediate release, but it would have been temporary, connected with time. Jesus had the eternal view. He knew the Big Plan of God. He was orchestrating the ultimate solution. He didn't rescue His beloved friend, relative and co-worker in His kingdom. People misunderstood and criticized Him because He seemed to be sitting on His hands. Neither did Jesus raise John from the dead, although He could have.

When Jesus heard of the life-threatening illness of His good friend Lazarus, He could have healed him even by long-distance as He did in another case. He didn't. Again Jesus was misunderstood and criticized because He seemed to be sitting on His hands. However, Jesus had the eternal perspective. He knew the Big Plan of God. He was orchestrating the eternal solution. His good friend died, but Jesus performed a greater act than healing. He raised Lazarus from the dead, illustrating and teaching a spectacular truth. It wasn't a *permanent* resurrection. Eventually, Lazarus died again.

Sometimes Jesus "healed all who came to Him." On other occasions He didn't. He could have delivered Himself from death on the cross, but He didn't. God didn't deliver Him either. It seemed as if God was sitting on His hands while His only begotten Son died. God had a Big Plan. He was orchestrating eternal salvation for sinful mankind.

If God heals me now, instantly, it would still be temporary. If God wills to take me through the surgical adventure and heal me in that way, it would also be temporary. My body is mortal and subject to eventual human death. The question is, what will bring glory to God in my present experience?

In the case of the man born blind, Jesus declared that God deliberately allowed his infirmity so that He could display the glory of God. I must leave the decision to God alone whether He will be glorified through my instant healing or surgery, followed by recovery or not . . . or no healing and my soon entrance into heaven. God has a Big Plan. He is working out the best possible solution.

I'm absolutely sure *God is not sitting on His hands!* On the contrary, He holds me in His hands! ◆

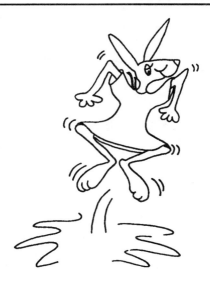

My Personal Workout

1. What are some possible sources of illness other than the consequence of one's own wrong doing, indulgences, abuse or neglect?

2. Do I truly believe God is in control of what is happening to me, or do I feel I am in the clutches of random happenings or a target of Satan's attacks?

3. What does God's Word tell me about God's sovereignty? Does the devil have limited or unlimited power?

4. What is my most important question related to my own illness?

5. What spiritual and human resources do I have as a Christian?

6. Do I believe God *does* still heal today and that He *can* heal me? On what Scriptures do I base my faith?

7. Do I insist on supernatural healing in response to my faith?

8. Am I willing to accept whatever God determines is best for my good and for his glory? Will I still trust Him if He doesn't heal me? What are my struggles regarding this possibility?

9. Why does God sometimes refuse or delay healing in spite of our prayers, the prayers of others, and the exercise of our faith?

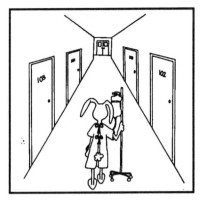

Chapter 4

No Answer

Why doesn't God pick up the phone? I keep calling Him. *I would like to hear God's voice with my own ears.*

The Bible recorded that God spoke to His people. If I called, He promised to answer me. "In the day of my trouble I shall call upon Thee, for Thou wilt answer me" (Psalm 86:7). It *is* my day of trouble. I don't get a busy signal, just no answer.

The Bible declared that God is an *ever-present* help in time of trouble. (Psalm 46:1) Why does He seem *never-present* when I'm in trouble? "For He stands at the right hand of the needy" (Psalm 109:31). I'm desperately needy, but I don't see Him anywhere around.

Either there is something wrong with God or with

me. I know the problem can't be with Him, so I guess it must be with me. If God seems distant when He assures me He is close, how do I recognize His closeness?

I feel like Martha when she complained to Jesus, "If you had been here, my brother would not have died." I feel that if God had been here, my calamity would not have happened. If only He would *say something* to assure me He's in control, I could go through this more patiently.

Charles Stanley identifies with that dilemma in his book, *How to Handle Adversity:*

> One of the most frustrating things about Christianity is that our God is oftentimes so quiet. . . . I would like a little response. Anything would be fine, and yet He is silent. The strange thing is that I am acutely aware of God's silence when I need Him the most. . . . [But] God's silence is in no way indicative of His activity or involvement in our lives. *He may be silent, but He is not still.* We assume that since we are not hearing anything He must not be doing anything.
>
> We judge God's interest and involvement by what we see and hear. . . . So what am I supposed to do in the meantime? The answer to that is simple, though it is not necessarily easy. Trust God. . . . If you are not going to trust God, what are you going to do? . . . When have you ever turned your back on God's plan and come out a winner? . . . When God is silent, you have only one reasonable option—trust Him, hang in there and wait on Him. He may be quiet, but He has not quit on you.[1]

Am I doing my part?

When I think more rationally, I can't say God is silent just because I can't hear Him *right now.* God spoke in the past through His Word and through the experiences of His people. He speaks to me through clear impressions and guidance. His voice is still as close to my ear as the open pages of the Bible are to my eyes.

Why should I insist on *some new word* from God? He *has already spoken* and never reneged on His promises or His faithfulness. It's time for me to go to the spiritual freezer and take out what I have stored there for my time of need.

God's promises will taste as good today as when they were fresh. I'll thaw them out in my microwave of prayer and nourish myself.

If I tuned my hearing aid to God's frequency, I could probably hear Him saying, as He said before, "He who has ears to hear, let him hear."

Looking back on my spiritual journey, it makes sense to travel a proven route based on a Scriptural principle. "Let us therefore draw near with confidence to the throne of grace, that we may receive mercy and may find grace to help in time of need" (Hebrews 4:16). If I don't feel God near me, nevertheless *I'm supposed to draw near to Him.* I will then find His mercy and grace and enjoy a sense of His presence when I need it.

To practice the presence of God I must walk continually with Him. *I'm never out of His presence* whether I feel it or not. I am in His "ever-present" circle; I shouldn't bounce in and out of it, struggling to stay close to Him. If I listen to Him on a moment-by-moment basis, my ears are always tuned to His frequency. "Nevertheless I am continually with Thee. . . . But as for me, the nearness of God is my good" (Psalm 73:23,28).

God fulfills His promises to me when I walk in His way. It's a simple matter of putting my ear where His promises are.

Cart before the horse

How silly to think of a cart pulling a horse! First things first. Things of greater importance should take priority.

Healing is big on my mind. Nevertheless, more important than my physical healing is my spiritual wholeness and the assurance of forgiveness for my sins. The horse pulls the cart, of course. In the third verse of Psalm 103, David harnesses the horse properly. "[The Lord] Who *pardons* all your iniquities; [then] Who *heals* all your diseases." First things first.

If God heals me of my illness but doesn't forgive my sins, I'm still sick or un-whole. At best, physical healing is a *Band-Aid*. The time will come in my mortal life when doctors can no longer patch up my body because it's made of earthly stuff. I am "an earthen vessel," a clay pot. However, the healing of my soul and spirit, that *permanent* part of me, consists of eternal stuff. The forgiveness of my sins prepares me for everlasting life *after* my mortal body gives out.

God offers me *pardon*. He doesn't overlook my sin or excuse me. Pardon is for someone who has indeed committed a transgression but is absolved or acquitted *after* he is found guilty. Christ took my sin upon Himself so that I don't have to suffer the consequences.

He has not dealt with us according to our
sins, nor rewarded us according to our iniquities. For as high as the heavens are above the
earth, so great is His lovingkindness toward
those who fear Him. As far as the east is from
the west, so far has He removed our transgres-
sions from us. (Psalm 103:10-12)

To prepare for God to heal me physically, if that
is His will, I need His total forgiveness. I should have no
known or unconfessed sin in my life. Whatever happens
to my body after that is really inconsequential.

Once to die

Obviously, there *is* "sickness unto death," a term
Jesus used in the gospels. "It is appointed for men to die
once and after this comes judgment" (Hebrews 9:27).
The time will come when I cannot postpone my appointment with God—nor should I want to—because of the joy
that awaits me in His presence. I will have to keep my
appointment. No further physical rescue will be possible.
God created my body and its functions only for earthly
life. They will wear out or succumb to disease, illness,
accidents or the natural aging process. Early or late, that
time will come to me as it comes to every human being
and living creature on this planet.

The only exception to this universal law is if we are
alive when Christ returns. Such a miraculous, end-time
appearance by Jesus will mean that Christians living at
that time will escape natural death. *It is possible!* (1
Thessalonians 4:13-18) Otherwise, I am terminal, and
so is everyone else.

If I could be sure my particular illness *is* unto death, I would accept it. When that time comes, I will need His *dying grace,* not His *healing grace.* His timing will be perfect although I may dispute it from my human perspective. My sovereign, omniscient God predestines my time of death.

The disciple John used intriguing terminology in John 21:19, "Now this He [Jesus] said signifying *by what kind of death he [John] would glorify God. . . ."* When that time comes, I pray that my death will glorify God.

As He has given abundant grace for my living, He will generously provide grace for dying. My dying may not be graceful, humanly speaking. *Death is not a friend. Death is an enemy.* (1 Corinthians 15:26) Physical death is the Great Separator from all things familiar to me and absence from those I love. But death is an enemy that Jesus already overcame for us at His resurrection. I don't have to conquer it again. Jesus triumphed over death. "For I am convinced that . . . death . . . shall [not] be able to separate us from the love of God, which is in Christ Jesus our Lord" (Romans 8:38-39).

Christ is in me, I am in Christ, and my "life is hidden with Christ in God," (Colossians 3:3). Since I already have eternal life, I should more accurately describe death as *continuing my eternal life* without interruption. Hallelujah! Where is death's sting?

Just thought I'd ask . . .

There is also sickness *not* unto death, but "in order that the works of God might be displayed in him" (John 9:3). Other versions of the Bible translate that passage "to demonstrate the power of God," "to illustrate it," and "so that God's power might be seen at work in him."

Until I'm sure of my joyful divine death sentence, I'll be bold and ask for a reprieve, like Jesus did, that "*if possible* this cup could pass from me." But I must immediately follow this request, as Jesus did, and as C.H. Spurgeon expressed it, "Spread your petition before God and then say 'Thy will be done.' The sweetest lesson I have learned in God's school is to let the Lord choose for me."

Our Father who is in heaven generously wants to give what is good to those who ask Him. (Matthew 7:12) So I dare to make my request because the Lord invited me:

> And everything you ask in prayer, believing, you shall receive. (Matthew 21:22)

> Ask and it shall be given to you; seek, and you shall find; knock, and it shall be opened to you. For everyone who asks receives, and he who seeks finds, and to him who knocks it shall be opened. (Matthew 7:7,8)

> You do not have because you do not ask. You ask and do not receive, because you ask with wrong motives. (James 4:2,3)

I must measure my motives against the selfish criteria explained by James in the verses that follow the above passage in James chapter four. Then, having asked boldly, specifically, humbly and with sincere motives to please and serve God, I leave my request to His perfect decision.

> **How big must my faith muscles be before
> God answers prayer? I flex mine and they seem
> as skinny as a chicken's.**

God doesn't say that I have to pump iron to get extraordinary faith before He hears and answers me. I'm hanging onto his mustard seed illustration. (Matthew 17:20)

To say "Thy will be done" is not to save God's face in case He doesn't want to grant my request. God doesn't need me to shield Him or excuse Him by making only generic requests. I believe "Thy will be done" is the line I draw after listing my requests, the line that recognizes God's wisdom and sovereignty.

No Answer

Dig in, hide or be rescued?

I have now come to the place of no-nonsense faith. These expressions may be worn, but still good for retreading: *This is where the rubber meets the road. My back is to the wall. I am between a rock and a hard place.* But I prefer to say, "between The Rock [Christ Jesus] and a hard place." Any problem that presses you closer to Jesus is your friend.

Apparently God doesn't always respond the same when we cry to Him for relief from whatever affliction or distress we are suffering. David says of God, "The Lord is my *rock* and my *fortress* and my *deliverer*" in Psalm 18:2. Those three titles describe characteristics of the Lord's working in our lives and are similarly grouped in several other references.

Sometimes God is a *Rock* for me to stand securely on, to hang on to. He wants me to dig in and endure my problem or my infirmity. In that case, I must learn to live with it as Paul did after God showed him it was for his highest good not to be free from a particular affliction. Deep water may surround the rock, but we won't get our feet wet. It may be a single large rock in the middle of a desert like I saw when I traveled in Egypt. We are refreshed in "the shadow of a mighty rock within a weary land" as the hymn writer testifies. The Rock is God Himself. The Scriptures are full of Rock promises. There is a time to "cling to the Rock that is higher than I" and let the storms of life rage on around us.

Sometimes God provides a *Fortress,* a refuge to run to, a safe place in which to hide for a time. When we are well-protected in God's fortress, the Lord deflects the fiery darts the wicked one aims at us. I am not a coward if I run to a refuge God provides and nestle under the shadow of His wings. There is a time to retreat to a fortress. "A mighty fortress is *our God.* . . ."

Sometimes God is our *Deliverer.* He decides to send His angelic rescue squad. It may be deliverance from the physical affliction into restored health and strength. Sometimes it is merciful deliverance from pain and infirmity by being ushered into His glorious presence. Physical death does not mean God didn't heal us or failed to answer prayer or denied our prayer. It is ultimate healing and refreshing release, a rescue from imperfect mortality and a transport to eternal immortality. It is God's triumphant promotion.

"There is an appointed time for everything. And a time for every event under heaven . . . a time to live . . . and a time to die" (Ecclesiastes 3:1,2). It's a good idea to leave the time and all the options to God.

The Lord may heal me of this affliction entirely, partially or temporarily. His name is *Jehovah-Rapha,* "the Lord who heals." (Exodus 15:26) Whether He heals me or not, I struggle with the question: Why did God heal someone else and not me? Or why did God heal me and not someone else? If I am the one healed, I should not feel proud and favored above others. If God does not heal me, I should not feel like a second-class citizen or think that God ignored or refused my request.

No matter how it turns out, my response should be daily, implicit trust in God. His grace *is* sufficient for me. Not *will be*, or *could be*, or *should be*, but God's grace *is* sufficient for me! (2 Corinthians 12:9)

Tap on the shoulder

If someone wants to get my attention, he may try several ways. He may call my name or motion to me. If he's close enough, he may tap me on the shoulder. Generally I won't ignore that gesture. I'll turn to see what my friend wants.

God uses various means to get our attention. He speaks through blessings, but unfortunately most of us don't listen as intently as when He speaks through adversity. He gets our attention through broken toys or broken dreams. Sometimes through misfortunes, failures or disappointments. Ignoring God's signals is hazardous to my spiritual health.

Perhaps I have been flying high on my own, busy and preoccupied with ordinary pursuits of life like family affairs, career, relationships, personal plans, goals and schedules—even ministry. Without realizing, I may have drifted from the priority of eternal concerns.

Charles Stanley brings out another aspect of God's attempt to get our undivided attention. God may not necessarily want to correct something in us, but to arouse and incite us to a deeper stage of maturity.

> We are not talking about a believer who has grown spiritually insensitive or who is running from God. This principle applies to those who are committed to doing the will of God. It presupposes a desire to grow. . . . What I am referring to are things such as character development, discernment, and the surrender of rights and possessions. These are areas of the spiritual life that take a lifetime to develop. . . . Only weeds and toadstools pop up overnight.
>
> Often we are unaware [of areas of immaturity]. So God sees fit to allow a little adversity into our lives to motivate us to do some self-examination. . . . It is not the kind of spiritual growth we look forward to or pray for. . . . But during those times we make the greatest strides forward in our relationship with God and others. . . . If we allow God to reveal all He wishes to reveal, permanent change takes place.[2]

Troubles, struggles and problems are a normal part of the curriculum in my classroom of the Christian life, although I would just as soon play hookey from such lessons. The Scriptures tell me that I shouldn't be surprised when The Teacher schedules tests. God plans them to nurture my spiritual growth and maturity. His will for me is not to *groan and bear* them, or even to *grin and bear* them. He wants me *to rejoice in them.*

Afflictions of one sort or another come to me as a Christian with redemptive meaning. God has my good in mind when He brings me through them. I may appropriately ask God *why* in the spirit of sincere *inquiry*, but not with a complaining, whining, rebellious attitude. My question should not challenge His sovereign actions. If God does not explain the reason right on the spot, I must be patient. He will make it clear later or in Eternity.

Why did You tap me on the shoulder this time, Lord? If I were an unbeliever, You would be inviting me to come to You. Since I am already one of Your own, You invite me to come closer, grow deeper and grow up! So my prayer is, "Make me know Thy ways, O Lord; teach me Thy paths. Lead me in Thy truth and teach me" *(Psalm 25:4,5).*

Who claims this body?

Whatever is going wrong in my human body, whether failed health or damage to my body from an accident, takes place on *God's* property. This flesh isn't really *my* body; it is *the Lord's.* What a different perspective this puts on my illness!

I've sung, "The Lord is in His holy temple" while visualizing God's presence in our church service. However, in this church age, a *building* is not God's "sanctuary" in the biblical sense. *People* are God's sanctuary—people who have accepted Jesus Christ. A church auditorium is where "living sanctuaries" gather at certain times to praise and worship God. *I* am God's property. *I* am His sanctuary.

The Bible tells me, "For we are the temple of the

living God" (2 Corinthians 6:16). "Do you not know that you are a temple of God, and that the Spirit of God dwells in you? . . . for the temple of God is holy, and that is what you are" (1 Corinthians 3:16, 17). When he spoke of the temple being destroyed, John explained, "But He [Jesus] was speaking of the temple of His body."

In the words of one of my favorite gospel songs:

> Lord, make me a sanctuary
> pure and holy, tried and true.
> Purify me from within
> fill me with your Holy Spirit
> and take away all my sin.
> Then I'll be
> a living sanctuary for you.

In Old Testament days, the Lord God dwelled *with* His people at certain times, and His power and Spirit came *upon* them. But He did not live *in* them. God's people worshiped Him at altars they built for sacrifices as He commanded them. Later God manifested His holy presence in the innermost room of the Tabernacle called "The Holy of Holies" where only the High Priest could go once a year. Still later, people worshiped God in the Temple built by King Solomon.

When Jesus came to earth as God's Son, He was at last the full expression of God revealed to men. When Jesus left the earth for heaven, He promised to send the Holy Spirit to those who believed in Him, and He declared that He would *live in* each of their bodies. That makes *each believer, including me,* a sanctuary of the Holy Spirit.

So what? That means that my illness, the abnormality, whatever it is, is *not separate* from the Lord. Isn't that awesome? That truth should change my outlook as I suffer the discomforts of tests, biopsies, surgery, pain or whatever my complaint is. It is all happening *to His property!*

Christ is in me by His Spirit; He never leaves me; His miraculous power heals me as I cooperate with the skill of physicians, the advancements of medicine and the natural recuperative powers God built into my human body.

"The Lord *is in* His holy temple." That's *me!* He is the one who claims my body!

Tentin' on the ol' campground

My body talks to me. By its creaks and groans, its sags and wrinkles, its increasing complaint of overload—and this current illness—my body lets me know that some of its parts are wearing out. My mortality shows.

I'm a perishable container of clay. Second Corinthians chapters four and five post a notice that as a human being I am an earthen vessel. My body is for temporary use. That's the bad news. Or is it?

As a Christian, the good news is that God has a reason for allowing me to be so fragile—so that "everyone can see that the glorious power within must be from God and is not our own" (2 Corinthians 4:7 TLB). When I manage to live victoriously in this transient body, all the credit goes to God, not to me.

Paul said that "our outer nature is wasting away." Other versions translate that phrase, "our bodies are dying," and "our outer nature suffers decay," and "our outward man perishes." Visits to the dentist, doctor, chiropractor or the beauty salon underscore that prognosis.

My body is only a tent for my use on this planet. If I am to have surgery, it is for maintenance repairs to my deteriorating tent.

When I was born, my human body clock started ticking toward countdown. Early in life my brain cells began to diminish—happy thought! Sooner than I want to admit, muscle tone and bone structure started downhill. Gravity kicks in. God didn't design us to hang around on earth very long.

Medical science races to devise "spare parts" for organs that no longer function as they should. Nevertheless, there is a limit to such earthly body shop repair. Certain parts of me will eventually break down, run down and wear out. I can't become an entirely bionic person.

My Creator-God planned the whole marvelous scenario! When Jesus Christ left this earth in His resurrected body, He said He was going to prepare our permanent living quarters elsewhere. Since I belong to Him, I've punched in my reservation already. He promised to turn my fragile earth-body into *a new model* suited for living in His supernatural kingdom.

What does this mean in my present physical distress? In this life I should *expect* broken and worn and diseased body parts. No surprise. We can temporarily patch whatever we can: fillings for our teeth (or porcelain replacements), hairpieces, heart bypasses, prosthetic limbs, hip sockets, lens implants, pacemakers and removal of lumps and bumps and growths that shouldn't be there. But what really excites me are the wonderful surprises ahead in heaven after my body parts entirely give out on earth.

Beside the highway I saw an encouraging construction sign that applies spiritually too: *"Temporary inconvenience, permanent improvement."* I may be on my way to some temporary inconvenience in the hospital body shop. But—no big deal, right? ◆

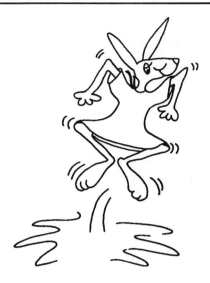

My Personal Workout

1. To what degree do I sense God's presence in my situation, or does He seem far off and silent?

2. Am I doing my part to "hear" Him? What conditions should I fulfill?

3. Has God proven faithful to me in the past? At what specific times? Therefore what can I expect of Him in this new situation?

4. Am I sure God has forgiven my sins? On what basis? Do I have any unconfessed sin about which God is dealing with me? Might that hinder my healing? According to 1 John 1:9 what can I do about my sin?

5. If my illness is terminal, am I sure I will go to heaven when I die? On what Scriptures do I base this assurance?

6. When the apostle Paul wrote about his impending death in Philippians 1:23, where did he say he would go and how soon did he expect to arrive? Did he consider this better or worse than living on earth?

7. Which of the three aspects of God—Rock, Fortress or Deliverer—is uppermost in my experience right now?

8. When we pray "if it be Thy will," is that a lack of faith? Why or why not? How does it reflect my humility, obedience and God's sovereignty?

9. For what reason might God be trying to gain my attention through this illness?

10. What difference does it make whether or not I recognize God's ownership of and responsibility for my physical body? What new perspective does this give me?

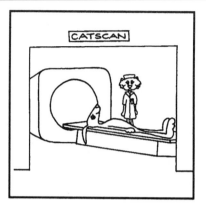

Chapter 5

Am I Finished?

Some people headed for surgery or suffering an illness try to avoid thinking deep, serious thoughts. They hunker down in their bunkers like Iraqi soldiers did in the heat of the Persian Gulf battle. They try not to face serious issues. They force themselves to think and talk about trivial, superficial things. That is a valid coping mechanism, of course.

I prefer grappling with the hard questions up front. Delay only postpones dealing with reality.

Some people wear a button that pleads, "Please be patient; God isn't finished with me yet." That's comforting, but it also makes me feel uneasy: Could I, after all, *be finished* with my life? Suppose I've run out of God's assigned time on earth for me?

I wrestle with words like "finished, completed, fulfilled." Life seems to be all about accomplishment, achievement, realization and successful attainment. But

I'm not *finished* yet. No matter how old I am, I don't feel that I've completed all my plans and fulfilled my dreams. If my life were over now, I would feel like a discontinued item, concluded, terminated. However, I would not be "done" in the sense of having "finished" all I hoped to do or be. I'm obsessed with my own plans, my doings. I know I don't need to accumulate merits *to attain* eternal life. God freely gives me that in response to my faith in Jesus Christ. *After* my eternal destiny is assured, God wants me to follow His plan for my life and no longer put my ambitions as priorities. But I have a problem: my mapped-out *personal* goals dangle like loose ends under the weaving of my life. I look at my life from the underside. God looks at it from above, from the perspective of eternity. He sees the finished design, His perfect plan.

The length of my life seems important to me, but God is not bound to time. That boggles my mind. *I could be finished with God's assignment for me and not know it!* My personal, unachieved goals may be beside the point—God's point. I need to correct my thinking to align with God's promises:

> The Lord will accomplish what concerns me; Thy lovingkindness, O Lord, is everlasting; Do not forsake the works of Thy hands. (Psalm 138:8)

> I will cry to God Most High, to God who accomplishes all things for me. (Psalm 57:2)

> For we are His workmanship, created in

Christ Jesus for good works, which God prepared beforehand, that we should walk in them. (Ephesians 2:10)

For I am confident of this very thing, that He who began a good work in you will perfect it until the day of Christ Jesus. (Philippians 1:6)

It is *God's responsibility,* not mine, to accomplish what concerns me. I am His work. Would He *terminate* my life before *He* is done? Cut it short earlier than He eternally planned it? Of course not. What He began He will finish and He will do it in His time. Jesus is the Alpha and the Omega, the beginning and the end. "[Christ] shall also confirm you to the end" (1 Corinthians 1:8).

My puny ambitions may not fit into His eternal design for the days and years of my life. His plans involving me were "prepared beforehand" with my name on the assignment. I accept that! What a fantastic thought! God doesn't expect me to be successful in the same way the world looks at success. He calls me to be faithful to His plan.

So, not to worry! God has His hands on the steering wheel of my life. He holds the stopwatch. I shouldn't call my illness *life-threatening.* God isn't threatening to cut me short. It is Satan who tries to intimidate me with the abortion of my days, but God won't allow it *until He is finished* with that which concerns me.

As I let down those sure anchors from His Word, they will keep my fragile boat from rocking or capsizing with fear and apprehension!

Comprehensive coverage

I've suddenly become intensely interested in my neglected file folder labeled "Health Insurance." Neglected because I've been incredibly strong and healthy most of my life. I discover that insurance companies limit the number of days they'll pay for a patient's care in the hospital, and they list many exclusions and limitations. I see a whole lot of small print and double talk.

Nevertheless, good news! I discover that I'm eligible to receive *unlimited lifelong care* from the Lord! That beats the best of insurance plans. God's policy in Psalm 30:5 promises, "His favor is for a lifetime." God's care for me will never run out. No age limit or exclusions for preexisting conditions—no restrictions—all the way to the end of my earthly life. That sure sounds great!

Nevertheless, I discovered something even better: "His lovingkindness is *everlasting*." I dived into Psalm 118 and highlighted all 26 times the psalmist repeated that marvelous promise. It echoes throughout Scripture. That convinced me that the Lord means just what He says. *Lifetime care* may be wonderful, but *everlasting care* from the Lord goes way over the top.

Health insurance may run out, they may cancel our car insurance, Social Security may go defunct and pension plans may collapse. A Wall Street crash may wipe out our savings and investments, and the D.M.V. may suspend our license to drive. We may not be able to buy life insurance, and hurricanes or earthquakes may destroy all that we have in the world.

Such things can happen to any of us—Christians and non-Christians alike. We may come to the end of our rope in any number of ways in days ahead, including losing our physical health. Still, *"His lovingkindness is everlasting!"*

The cherry on top of the whipped cream is the promise of Jesus, "Lo, I am with you *always*, even to the end of the age" (Matthew 28:20). The Amplified Bible extends the meaning: "I am with you all the days—perpetually, uniformly and on every occasion—to the [very] close *and* consummation of the age." That means into eternity, because Jesus promised, "I go to prepare a place for you, that where I am, there you may be also." God's comprehensive coverage gives me security that the world can never guarantee.

Thank You, Lord, for the assurance that whatever is ahead of me in this surgical adventure, Your life care will never run out, nor will You cancel it if I use it too often. Praise You for Your everlasting lovingkindness!

Safety net

I finally know how potentially serious my illness is. A second and third medical opinion confirmed it. My first impulse is to withdraw, to isolate myself. I'm not contagious, of course, but I want to hide in a corner and not tell anyone. I want to handle this thing myself, to put my hands over my ears, shut my eyes and assume the fetal position "till the storm passes by," or until the medical community stops shooting surprise "scud" missiles at me. I want to escape to my sealed room, as Israeli families did when the wailing siren sounded during Iraqi attacks.

My wailing siren screams danger. The "scud" missile is on its scary trajectory: *they have scheduled my surgery!*

The big battle is still ahead, and I don't have "Patriot missiles" to shoot back and intercept the "scud." I feel that I am at the mercy of my predicament. That's my first response. My second is more sane. I realize I should do just the opposite: come out of my sealed room and count my incredible assets. I have an enormous supply of weapons and ammunition and a sophisticated, state-of-the-art defense system. I have an immense stockpile of both spiritual reserves and human resources.

God is my Command and Control. I can be courageous and daring if I follow His orders implicitly. He is familiar with the whole battlefield. God has already done the R. & D. for the campaign to come. He has been preparing me for years to engage in spiritual field combat, training me in spiritual warfare. I'll fly His flag, keep my head down and keep cool.

I have a potential defense and offense network of family, friends and prayer partners ready to back me up with whatever spiritual supply I need. Therefore, I should tell them about my pending battle, call them, write them, alert them to my need. My human tendency is to resist doing that and go through this unknown adventure quietly alone. As a Christian, I hope I know better.

Bearing one another's burdens expresses the fellowship, empathy, compassion and understanding of my brothers and sisters in Christ. (Galatians 6:2) God isn't pleased when the members of His body, the church, try to go it alone. No problem is too trivial. No problem is too serious to hide. I should give others the opportunity to help me bear my burden.

Therefore, I call on them, not for sympathy but for support. God is recruiting an entire battalion of spiritual military personnel in full spiritual combat gear to back me up. When I'm weak, terrified and apprehensive on the front line, *I'm not alone.*

As awesome, wonderful and comforting as it is to know that many friends are holding a net of prayer under me, my greatest support is that *Jesus is praying for me!* By implication, the entire High Priestly prayer of Jesus in John 17 is for me. The authority of verse 20 includes me. When Jesus prayed, it was not for His disciples alone, but "for those also who believe in Me through their word." *That's me.* As Jesus assured Peter, "I have prayed for you that your faith fail not," so I believe His intercession reaches me.

The Holy Spirit intercedes for me too! "The Spirit Himself intercedes for us with groans that words cannot express. And he who searches our hearts knows the mind of the Spirit, because the Spirit intercedes for the saints in accordance with God's will" (Romans 8:26,27 NIV).

Praise God that "underneath are His everlasting arms," (Deuteronomy 33:27) and underneath I also have "the safety net" of my praying friends, my praying Lord and the praying Holy Spirit! I'm counting on these marvelous resources as I walk the tightrope of surgery and whatever is to follow.

Imaging center

My first appointment is at the Imaging Center, an antiseptic modern building with a friendly potted-plant reception room and bustling, white-clad staff. I am here to let them expose and display in detail "all that is within me" by a CT "CAT" scan and x-rays. I have a spot, an "unidentified (non)flying object" within. The surgeon needs a precise, detailed location on film before he tries to remove it.

I keep reminding myself that because I belong to the Lord He plans all that happens to me. "Bless the Lord, O my soul, and *all that is within me*" (Psalm 103:1). That must include the abnormality inside and whatever is to be done about it.

The CAT scan first sees and then reveals the deepest reaches of my physical being without cutting me open. Modern technology is incredible! It will see my "spot" and give my surgeon measurements of its density, size, shape and anything else he needs to know.

The radiologist and technicians at the Imaging Center see what's in "my temple," as the Lord calls my body. But the machine won't display Christ, although He is there within me, and is more real than what they see. God said that He is there " . . . through His Spirit in the inner man; so that Christ may dwell in your hearts through faith" (Ephesians 3:16,17). He transforms me into His image through the circumstances He allows in my life—like this unexpected surgery.

Search me, [CAT scan me] O Lord, and know my heart; try me and know my anxious thoughts; and see if there be any hurtful way in me, and lead me in the everlasting way. (Psalm 139:23,24)

Yes, "image me" Lord. If I have some unconfessed sin or rebellious spot in me, that is worse than if I have a physical abnormality that needs to be removed. I confess it now. Remove the abnormality of my sin by Your spiritual surgery.

Lord, I want to be "without spot or wrinkle or any such thing" (Ephesians 5:27). I want to be a part of Your bride, whole and clean and forgiven. Only if I have "nothing between my soul and the Savior" can I peacefully enter the experience You have, in Your love, set before me.

Friendly fire

The Persian Gulf war brought the intriguing term "friendly fire" to our attention again. At first the two words seem contradictory. To be "under fire" sounds hostile, deadly, not friendly. Friendly fire comes from one's own military buddies in the heat and confusion of battle, not from the enemy.

The surgeon's knife cuts a friendly incision. God brings me through a special kind of friendly fire. It's not for my hurt, but for my healing. God doesn't do it accidentally but on purpose as part of His design for my life.

Fire can be harmful when it burns good flesh. Fire can be beneficial and healing when it cauterizes unhealthy flesh. Fire destroys combustible material, but it also refines silver and gold. A silver refining furnace, for instance, is a scorching place because of the intensely high temperatures needed for the process. I've heard that a worker watches the vats of liquid silver very carefully. The moment he sees his face reflected in the silver, he knows the fire is hot enough to remove the refined silver.

When we finally reflect the Lord's image in our adverse situation, the Lord declares "Enough is enough" and delivers us from the furnace. 2 Corinthians 3:18 tells me about it from another angle. "But we all, with unveiled face beholding as in a mirror the glory of the Lord, are being transformed into the same image from glory to glory, just as from the Lord, the Spirit." God intends my illness and surgery, under His careful temperature control, to be refining experiences for me.

"And I will bring [them] through the fire, refine them as silver is refined, and test them as gold is tested. They will call on My name, and I will answer them; I will say, 'They are My people,' and they will say, 'The Lord is my God'" (Zechariah 13:9). I can either accept this experience as a positive process by which God purifies and perfects my life, or resist it and call it evil. God uses friendly fire to bring the genuine out of me. (1 Peter 1:6,7) I should not think of my trial as something out of the ordinary:

> Beloved, do not be surprised at the fiery ordeal among you, which comes upon you for your testing, as though some strange thing were happening to you; but to the degree that you share the sufferings of Christ, keep on rejoicing; so that also at the revelation of His glory, you may rejoice with exultation. (1 Peter 4:12,13)

Lord, I do want to "go for the silver." Better yet, "go for the gold" in the spirit of Olympic champions! The heat of the experience is no leisurely stroll through an air-conditioned mall, but it results in God's approval as He says, "She is My child." And I agree: "The Lord is my God." His promise should cancel all my fears:

> Do not fear, for I have redeemed you; I have called you by name; you are Mine! When you pass through the waters, I will be with you; and through the rivers, they will not overflow you. When you *walk through the fire,* you will not be scorched, nor will the flame burn you. For I am the Lord your God, The Holy One of Israel, your Savior. (Isaiah 43:1-3)

I can make it through that kind of friendly fire because God is my asbestos suit!

If I should *die* before I wake . . .

"Now I lay me down to sleep; I pray Thee, Lord, my soul to keep. If I should die before I wake, I pray Thee, Lord, my soul to take."

Perhaps they don't teach children that bedtime prayer anymore. A positive-thinking generation of parents may have decided that the thought of dying in one's sleep is not an appropriate prayer for a little child. The youngster may be scared to close his eyes!

I like to face reality head on, in advance if necessary, and then to go on living with a lighter heart. I make my dry runs, go through rehearsals, and then life doesn't take me greatly by surprise. A surgical tap on the shoulder orchestrated by God takes one through the ultimate dry run of dying.

No one has the option of staying permanently on planet Earth. There is no "Plan B." We are all terminal. Nevertheless, for the Christian, death is limited to the human, physically functioning body.

"If I should die before I wake. . . ." Well, I want to remind myself what the Bible teaches about "life after life."

Whenever my "step over" time comes, I'll doubtless leave personal plans, tasks, ambitions, dreams and ministry goals incomplete according to *my* limited, human opinion. I may not want to leave yet, although I'm not afraid of physical death. Jesus took "the sting" from it by His resurrection.

The Bible tells me that through my faith in Jesus Christ as my personal Savior, I'm already enjoying eternal life from the moment I was born again. Spiritually, *I'll never stop living.*

According to what I believe the Bible teaches, at the time my heart stops, my brain dies and my mortal, physical body ceases to function, my immortal spirit is released. It goes immediately into the presence of Christ, wherever He is. The Bible gives us comparatively few details about our "life after life." Nevertheless, Jesus told us enough to give us the assurance He is now "preparing a place for us." (John 14:1-6) I expect to be fully conscious in the presence of Christ, retain my identity and not go through any unconscious sleeping stage.

The Bible declares that God has a glorious plan for His people and for the whole physical world as we know it. In fact, a plan for the entire universe for all space and time. Therefore I don't need to fear the *unknown* because I personally *know* Him Who is in control of it. I believe Christians will enjoy "bushels of wonderful surprises" the moment they close their eyes for the last time on Earth and open them wide in the presence of Christ![1]

If I should *fly* before I wake . . .

According to what I believe the Bible teaches, I expect Jesus Christ to return to Earth at any moment, as He promised. That means He could appear while I'm in surgery! My body, although strapped to the O.R. table and hooked up to lots of monitors, would simply disappear as I joined living Christians all over the world to meet Christ in the air. (1 Thessalonians 4:13-18)

When Jesus appears above planet Earth, He will come to receive into heaven all those who belong to Him. This is not the same as Jesus' "Second Coming," which is a separate, later event. This prior appearance is specifically to take the church worldwide, His body, as He calls it, and the individual believers who are part of it, into His presence.

If I am a Christian and have already died when that happens, my human body, however long it was dead, will be resurrected and rejoin my immortal spirit, which was in the presence of Christ from my moment of death. Since the Bible says that "the dead in Christ shall rise first," all those who died as Christians throughout the ages will be raised a split second before Christians who may be alive on Earth then. I, with all Christians living or dead, will be immediately transported to heaven in the company of Christ. [2] Christians alive at that time will be the only ones to actually *skip the process of dying* and be immediately transformed into their immortal bodies. I believe the Bible teaches that we will all remain in heaven, or as Jesus called it, "My Father's House," for exciting scheduled events before we return with Jesus to Earth at His Second Coming. That will be the time when He will intervene in world affairs and stop the catastrophic wars which will be taking place. He will judge the nations and begin His thousand-year reign on this planet Earth.

The Bible states that we will come back to Earth with Him at His Second Coming and participate actively in His glorious reign on Earth until God establishes the New Heavens and New Earth to replace these present ones which will have passed away. Then we will continue to be with Christ forevermore. *This is a spectacular scenario I don't want to miss!*

If Jesus' sudden appearing should happen in the middle of my scheduled surgery, I would simply "split the scene" in "the twinkling of an eye," as the Bible describes it. So would my chief surgeon, a Christian believer, and probably some operating room personnel and hospital staff. The astonished ones left behind would have a bewildering time accounting for the disappearance of certain patients and medical personnel!

Another perk: I wouldn't have to worry about paying my hospital bill! ◆

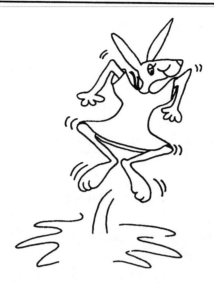

My Personal Workout

1. In what ways do I feel "not finished" with my life? How do I know from God's Word that He won't "cut me short" if I am a Christian?

2. Do I keep my problem to myself, or have I shared it with my family and friends to gain their support and prayers? What has been their response?

3. Read the Scriptures in "The Back of the Book" under the topics "Life After Life," and "Promises About the Future." Look them up in your own Bible to check their accuracy.

4. What terms are used in those Scripture verses to describe becoming a Christian? Am I sure I have I taken that step personally?

5. Describe what the Bible says will happen at the return of Christ: 1) to Christians who have already died, 2) to Christians living on Earth at that time.

6. How real to me is the anticipation and expectation of the return of Christ?

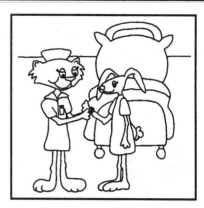

Chapter 6

No Wheeling
or Dealing

I don't mind driving on familiar roads, even coast to coast, if I have a good map. But when I try to find my way around China, I get a rush of adrenalin and my palms get cold and clammy. Why? No road maps in English!

Unprepared for a traumatic physical illness, I have the same sensations. I panic without a road map. My *first* surgical experience—no precedent. To say I have butterflies in my stomach is an understatement. It's more like a flock of frenzied poultry squawking and beating wings inside me. Yes, I'm "chicken." And I'm on the fringe of panic.

Some years ago my husband and I were returning

"on a slow boat to China" from ministry on the island of Hainan. The weather was stormy, waves choppy, and the small ship heaved up and down unmercifully. Both of us were green with seasickness. We climbed into our bunks so we wouldn't fall over with the constant lurching.

Beside the cracked mirror on the wall of our less-than-basic cabin a little sign both in Chinese and in "Chinglish" caught our attention because of its jumbled grammar. It read, *"If accident or incident occur, passengers are to keep calmness and obey what the Master say, instruct or arrange."* They capitalized the "M" in Master, obviously referring to the captain of that Oriental ship.

I'm trying to follow that advice today. Whatever happens in my life, whatever is ahead soon, I'm trying to "keep calmness," in the words of that crude little sign. No hysteria. No distress. Just "obey what the Master say."

My Master, my Lord, has plenty to say in His Word to assure me that He controls my life-ship and is the Commander of the waves that threaten to capsize it. The winds and the seas obey Him. I shouldn't lose my cool. Step by step, I should do what He "say, instruct or arrange."

My assurance comes from 1 Corinthians 10:13 (GNB):

> Every test that you have experienced is the kind that normally comes to people. But God keeps His promise, and He will not allow you to be tested beyond your power to remain firm; at the time you are put to the test, He will give you the strength to endure it, and so provide you with a way out.

God isn't singling me out for some rare experience. Anything ahead of me is "common to man" (and woman, of course). I just haven't traveled this road before.

If things get really rough, and I find myself in danger, I know my Master, my Captain, will provide a life preserver or a lifeboat, or He will calm the waves. "Thou dost rule the swelling of the sea; when its waves rise, Thou dost still them" (Psalm 89:9). Or maybe He will ask me to walk on the water like the disciple Peter. He calls the shots.

There's nothing worse than a swaying deck. The steady rail I cling to is "[The Lord] will never allow the righteous to be shaken" (Psalm 55:22). "Totter" is the marginal reading for "shaken."

I call Psalm 107 my seasick Psalm. I can't read it without feeling nauseous.

He spoke and raised up a stormy wind, which lifted up the waves of the sea. They rose up to the heavens, they went down to the depths; their soul melted away in their misery. They reeled and staggered like a drunken man, and were at their wits' end. Then they cried to the Lord in their trouble, and He brought them out of their distresses. He caused the storm to be still, so that the waves of the sea were hushed. Then they were glad because they were quiet; so He guided them to their desired haven. Let them give thanks to the Lord for His lovingkindness. (Psalm 107: 25-31)

I shouldn't be dismayed "whate'er betide," in the words of an old English hymn. "God will take care of you" (and me) whatever "accident or incident occur," as the little Chinglish notice instructed.

That creepy thing

I've dealt with my *panic*. Now I wrestle with another attacker—*anxiety*. It's quieter, but more sneaky. When I feel some creepy "unidentified flying object" (or a crawly one) on my arm or the back of my neck, I respond with an automatic, self-preservation reflex. I whisk it violently from me even before I think of mashing the insect, bug or fly to pulp. It doesn't belong on me and that's enough reason to get rid of it!

Anxiety is one of the most creepy things I know. When I brush it away, it's soon buzzing back intruding upon my emotions. It's never gone for good. I've been working through my questions and doubts and trying to make my way to faith and trust. But anxiety crawls back again and again.

There's only one way to deal with worry—God's way: "*Casting* all your anxiety (care, worry) upon Him because He cares for you" (1 Peter 5:7 ᵀᴸᴮ). I must fling worry away from me just as violently as I would a spider. Not only away from me, but I should cast it "upon Him," the Lord. Why? Because He told me I should, and I'm in God's intensive care.

I must not politely escort worry to the door with a pleasant "Come again at a more convenient time." At the first tickle or tingle of worry, I must get rid of it. I should never entertain it.

I don't share my problems with other people

unless I know they really care. But I don't hesitate to share them with the Lord. He *invites* me to roll my burdens on Him. Moreover, He has the authority to do something about them.

If I cast only part of my anxiety away, like flicking a bee from my arm after it has stung me, the stinger might remain. The poison can still enter my system. "Cast *all*. . . " I must give Him my whole burden. I must cast on the Lord not only the bulky, heavy furniture of obvious care, but all the weighty little things that may seem insignificant and petty.

Size is deceiving. A friend asked me to pick up a small piece of sparkling, slate-colored ore she uses as a paper weight. I nearly dropped it—it turned out to be lead and incredibly heavy. I realize that my worry backpack is full of such miniature but lead-heavy concerns that hamper my spiritual life during this crisis. They are really a burden.

In the same verse as above, the marginal reading of "your burden" is "what He has given you." What He is giving me right now is my illness. God will hold me up, support me, prop me up if necessary, so I won't fall flat on my face. He will carry my heavy burden.

Of course I'm tempted to worry as I face surgery. But I would be a poor example of God's trusting child if I gave in to it. Without a doubt God will take my worry burden upon Himself *if I do my part* and cast the cumbersome cargo upon Him.

Monster *Fear!*

Two opponents down and one to go. I've wrestled with *panic and anxiety*, now *fear* attacks me. I climb into the ring again. Fear comes charging at me in capital letters, in boldface and italics with an exclamation mark! Fear is a terrorist who has just heaved a hand grenade in my direction. My emotions are bleeding from the shrapnel. Fear has a stun gun that paralyzes my thinking.

It must have been Satan who threw the fear grenade at me because God's Word says *fear isn't from God.* I can't decide whether I'm afraid of death or the process of dying. Until now, dying always happened to someone else. I don't have to pinch myself to know this isn't a bad dream from which I'll awaken perspiring with relief. Death is real and so is fear.

> My heart is in anguish within me, and the terrors of death have fallen upon me. Fear and trembling come upon me; and horror has overwhelmed me. And I said, 'O that I had wings like a dove! I would fly away and be at rest.' Behold, I would wander far away, I would lodge in the wilderness. I would hasten to my place of refuge from the stormy wind and tempest. (Psalm 55:4-8)

That's how I feel. I'd like to say, "I'm outa here!" and escape the reality of what's to come. I don't have those wings about which David spoke, but the Lord is gracious to me. I do have "the shadow of Thy wings [under which] I will take refuge until destruction passes by. I will cry to God who accomplishes all things for me. He will send from heaven and save me" (Psalm 57: 1-3).

Fear is a four-letter word that towers in front of me like "Mr. Clean" in a detergent commercial on TV.

However, fear isn't antiseptic or harmless. Fear contaminates my whole being. It stands ten feet tall with massive, muscled-arms folded, legs apart. It reaches out and grabs my throat in a vice grip until I feel as if I'm choking. Fear presses against my chest giving me symptoms of suffocation.

God understands fear in His children. The Bible mentions fear 365 times. (Any significance in that number? One fear for each day of the year?) God sent angels to Earth repeatedly to announce, "Fear not!" Jesus used the same term often. Fear is common to mortal man, and to me, because I am helpless when I'm not in control. The antidote is clear:

> When I am afraid, I will put my trust in Thee, in God, whose word I praise. In God I have put my trust; I shall not be afraid. What can mere man do to me? (Psalm 56:3,4)

A note in my Bible introducing Psalm 27 reads "A Psalm of fearless trust in God." If I fear, I don't trust. My private world seems like a war zone. *Lord, my ammunition comes only from You!*

> The Lord is my light and my salvation; whom shall I fear? The Lord is the defense of my life; whom shall I dread? . . . Though a host encamps against me, my heart will not fear. Though war arises against me, in spite of this I shall be confident. (Psalm 27:1,3)

> For God has not given us a spirit of fear, but of power and of love and of a sound mind. (2 Timothy 1:7)

Since fear doesn't come with the Lord's return address, I know Satan sent it and I won't accept it. If I reject a piece of mail, I won't sign my name to receive it. I'll write on it "Refused. Return to sender."

Like a foot soldier, I camp on the battlefield of my illness. If I lift the flap of my tent to allow fear, like the proverbial camel, to stick its nose in, next it will nudge its foot into my tent. Soon the whole camel gets in my tent and takes over. Fear is like that. If you give it an inch, it crawls into your sleeping bag with you. When I first hear fear poking around my tent, that's the time I should chase it away with trust in God.

Double peace

Panic, anxiety, fear—they give birth to all the monsters in my *emotions* and my *mind*. If I successfully lasso my mind, my emotions are still flying out of control. How can I tie both of them securely to Jesus?

God thinks of everything. He *doubles* His promise: "And the peace of God, which surpasses all comprehension, shall guard *your hearts and your minds* in Christ Jesus" (Philippians 4:7). The security guard of God's peace will walk back and forth in front of my heart (my emotions) and my mind (my thoughts). His peace protects them and keeps them under His control.

My thoughts affect my emotions. Both affect my physical heart, blood pressure and my entire physical well-being. When I face surgery or proceed through recovery, I can't afford to have my emotions and mental state working against me.

God created me with emotions, with the ability to experience pain, sorrow, joy, pity, fear, resentment, anger—the whole gamut of human feelings. They are all prominent in such a crisis as this. Sometimes one or two surface at a time, sometimes it seems as if they all pile on me at once. I am painfully aware that they need to be under my Master's control.

The Lord tells me how I can secure His peace. The verse preceding the one above spells it out for me. "Be anxious for nothing but in everything by prayer and supplication with thanksgiving let your requests be made known to God" (Philippians 4:6).

First, I must not be anxious. I've already dealt with that, but I must fill the space left by "no anxiety" with two positives: "prayer and supplication." Supplication has the more intense meaning of a plea and an appeal. Panic prayer is something I can understand right now.

Then a third ingredient must enter the picture: "thanksgiving." Why should that be so important? Because I can look forward to receiving an answer from God in the present when I look back to recount His faithfulness in the past. He has answered me so often, and always cared for me. He delivered me time and again. That puts my present request in perspective.

His equation is now complete: "Prayer + supplication + thanksgiving = no anxiety."

If that's God's formula, then I know the clear path to no-anxiety and His peace. If I don't use His formula, God doesn't offer me any alternative.

Lord, help me do it Your way!

Peace—on condition

My mind still needs a little more attention before I can have peace. Most of God's promises are conditional. "Thou wilt keep him in perfect peace whose mind is stayed on Thee *because* He trusteth in Thee" (Isaiah 26:3). Apparently God can't keep me peaceful unless I take responsibility to anchor my mind on Him. His peace follows my obedient response.

If I don't keep my mind on God, it will go floating off like an untethered astronaut outside his space vehicle.

My mind is the fountain from which my anxieties bubble. When I allow my thoughts to run wild, they are not under the control of Christ. If I deliberately rein them in and bind them securely to Him, He *will* keep me in perfect peace. If that's what it takes, I must chase them with a butterfly net until I capture them. "Casting down imaginations, and every high thing that exalteth itself against the knowledge of God, and bringing into captivity every thought to the obedience of Christ" (2 Corinthians 10:5 KJV).

In the words of the hymn writer, "Stayed upon Jehovah, hearts are fully blessed, finding as He promised, perfect peace and rest." I must be strict with myself. I must deliberately, consciously think about Christ and fill my mind with words from Scripture. If I don't, my mind will slip into the anxiety cycle again.

My struggle never seems to be over. I must keep vigilant. Nevertheless, God is faithful each time I fulfill the condition to anchor my mind squarely on Him. Then I experience His peace. It's always available.

Cramming for the exam

A blood test revealed my dangerously low potassium level. The doctor prescribed massive doses of potassium for several days before surgery. He advised me to double my multivitamin intake, and to be sure I took enough iron. Apparently I need to be healthy so I can be sick! Likewise, I can't afford to be sick spiritually when I enter the hospital.

I must be able to say with the hymn writer, "It is well, it is well with my soul." A healthy spirit is essential if I want to make it through the ordeal and recover. According to God's Word, physical and spiritual health have some correlation. "Beloved, I pray that in all respects you may prosper and be in good health, *just as your soul prospers*" (3 John 2).

Normally, cramming for spiritual health and building spiritual stamina at the last minute would not be possible. When a soldier is sent into combat, it's too late to start training in boot camp. When you're thrown into deep water, the time for swimming lessons is over. A lazy, indifferent spiritual life and a remote relationship with the Lord reveal shallowness in a time of crisis.

Although I've walked with the Lord for a lifetime, I suddenly feel unprepared for this new crisis. I know I should be closer to the Lord. I'm taking too much for granted. To run on automatic in my Christian life is all too easy. I continually battle my inclination to self-reliance, although I know the Lord wants me to lean wholly on Him and not on my own understanding.

God is so gracious, so generous to stoop to my weakness and superficiality. He gives me emergency rations. He accepts a truly willing spirit for the deed done.

So I'm cramming anyway. I try to take large lumps of time to listen quietly to Him. I try to soak up Scripture promises as I flip the pages of my Bible. I search for relevant anchors to use in the weeks and months ahead.

This is something I *can* control. I can *determine* to repeat potent Bible promises over and over. I don't choose complicated, long verses because I expect to be functioning in crisis mode. I choose simple ones:

"Christ in you, the hope of glory" (Colossians 1:27).

"Thou wilt keep Him in perfect peace whose mind is stayed upon Thee, for he trusteth in Thee" (Isaiah 26:3).

"Peace I leave with you, My peace I give unto you. . . . Let not your heart be troubled, neither let it be afraid" (John 14:27).

A phrase or verse of a hymn may help calm my mind. "Whatever my lot, Thou hast taught me to say, 'It is well, it is well with my soul.'"

"Jesus, I am resting, resting, in the joy of what Thou art."

"Stayed upon Jehovah, hearts are fully blessed, finding as He promised, perfect peace and rest."

I read many verses into my cassette tape recorder to take to the hospital. I plan to listen to them through my stereo headset. During early stages of recovery I understand that I may not be able to read for very long at a time because my eyes won't focus and will tire. Nevertheless God's Word will still be more necessary than my food. I'll need to ingest His promises some way. I'll be able to listen to them without disturbing others. If I can only manage to push the "Play" button, I'll be O.K.

While I record the verses, I feast on the significance of them for my crisis. I sense the importance of "Let the word of Christ richly dwell within you, with all wisdom. . . ." (Colossians 3:16). I desperately need God's Word to build up my spirit, quiet me and reinforce my trust in Him.

I regret that I didn't memorize many more verses in the past. I feel so skinny in my soul. *Lord, have mercy on me.*

No wheeling or dealing

I can't do any wheeling or dealing with God. This is not like the television game show, "Let's Make a Deal." I can't see what's behind Door # 1, # 2 or # 3 in my life, and I can't trade anything I have to get the hidden contents. The game show contestants always hope that whatever is behind a particular door will be better or more valuable than what they bargain with. In reality, I have *nothing* with which to bargain.

**I can't "plea bargain." I have no right to ask
God to trade me health or healing for something
I can offer Him.**

I can't say, "God, if you'll just make me well, I'll give you this or that in my life." Or "I'll serve you all the days of my life, if you just get me through this crisis." Or "I'll never do such and such again, if only you'll do a miracle for me this time." God owns everything. He doesn't need anything I have. He is already managing my life from beginning to end. I stand empty-handed.

The only acceptable attitude is to prostrate myself before Him in surrender and confess, *"Lord, I am Yours, all Yours, no matter what. You have full rights of possession to order my life, my body and its condition and the length of my years. Whatever You decide, Lord, I worship You. I praise Your holy name. I have no higher court of appeal than Your Majesty."*

No ifs, ands or buts. I don't set the conditions. I accept God's decisions. With the hymn writer I declare, "Just as I am, without one plea . . . . O Lamb of God, I come! I come!" With Job I will stand upon my belief in the goodness of God: "Though He slay me, yet will I trust Him. . . ." (Job 13:15)

No way but through

I have come to the place where I can take no detours. No more scheduled tests, biopsies, x-rays, CAT scans, blood tests, medical consultations or second opinions to seek. No forks in the road, no turning back.

For His own perfect reasons, apparently God isn't going to deliver me from this surgical adventure. Therefore, He must have planned what I will go through. I can't escape it and should not try to squirm out of it. *There is no way but through.*

"Through" is an optimistic word, however. It implies that there is an exit, an "afterward." There is light at the end of the tunnel. For a surgery or illness, that outlet from the tunnel will either be: "It's over now; time for recovery," or "the liftoff" experience of death into the presence of Christ—an immediate, perfect healing and a new, immortal body. If my time on earth isn't over yet, recovery will probably be the more difficult outcome. The liftoff into God's presence would be easiest and the most joyful!

In either case, God has given me a checkbook full of marvelous "through" promises. He has already signed each one. I'm going to cash them as I need them. I can't overdraw the account since this is a God-planned experience. I'm eager to run to the bank with the first handful of Divine checks. Here's one of them:

Who shall separate us from the love of Christ? Shall tribulation, or distress, or persecution, or famine, or nakedness, or peril, or sword?. . . But in all these we overwhelmingly conquer through Him who loved us. For I am convinced that *neither death, nor life,* nor angels, nor principalities, nor things present, nor things to come, nor powers, nor height, nor depth, nor any other created thing, shall be able to separate us from the love of God, which is in Christ Jesus our Lord. (Romans 8:35,37-39)

I've been doing a countdown on the calendar . . . 10 days, 9, 8, 3—*tomorrow!* I try to look at it another way: next week at this time *it will all be over!* Or, a month from tomorrow I'll be having a one-month checkup. Or . . . by tomorrow night I might be with the Lord! I find new meaning in the verse, "So teach us to *number our days* that we may apply our hearts unto wisdom" (Psalm 90:12). To countdown to the event somehow gives me a little space to deal with my own emotions.

C.S. Lewis expressed it, "God whispers to us in our pleasures, speaks in our own conscience, but shouts in our pain: it is His megaphone to rouse a deaf world." Yes, to rouse *me,* if I have grown hard of hearing to His still, small voice.

My day in court

Finally, *tomorrow is my day in court!* I have cast myself on the mercy of God, the Judge of my spiritual Supreme Court. "Mercy" is the word to which I cling. My plea is based on my desire to live a little longer so I can glorify God on earth and finish some work He may still want me to do.

God, the Divine Judge, after reviewing the facts of my case, will hand down the decision. It will please Him if I accept it gladly rather than throwing a temper tantrum. *Mercy* may be God's decision. How happy I would be to have my surgery canceled! But I have added to my prayer, as Jesus did, "Nevertheless, not my will be done, but thine." God may get a lot more glory from having me go through the surgical experience than my escaping it.

In the apostle Paul's case, he called his "thorn in the flesh," whatever it was, "a messenger of Satan," although he still *called upon God* to rid him of it. Was it a physical ailment? Probably, but we don't know for sure. Paul certainly didn't want any part of it. He repeatedly, three deliberate times, asked God to remove it. Various translations use the words "besought, begged, called, invoked," that it be removed. God didn't remove it. It wasn't that God was mean about it, or didn't hear Paul. Obviously God had a better plan. Paul eventually realized God was using his affliction "to keep me from exalting myself." The bottom line for Paul should be the bottom line for me. Paul didn't get a *reprieve,* but God gave him sufficient *grace* to bear it.

But He said to me, My grace—My favor and loving-kindness and mercy—are enough for you, [that is, sufficient against any danger and to enable you to bear the trouble manfully]; for *My* strength *and* power are made perfect—fulfilled and completed *and show themselves most effective*—in [your] weakness. Therefore, I will all the more gladly glory in my weaknesses *and* infirmities, that the strength *and* power of Christ, the Messiah, may rest—yes, may pitch a tent [over] and dwell—upon me! (2 Corinthians 12:9, Amplified)

How descriptive! How awesome that God promises to *pitch a tent* of strength and power over me! I can just snuggle inside that shelter, that refuge, and *glory* in my infirmities. Yes, and *boast* about my weaknesses. That's what Paul recommended by example:

So for the sake of Christ, I am well pleased *and* take pleasure in infirmities . . . for when I am weak (in human strength), then am I [truly] strong—able, powerful in divine strength. (2 Corinthians 12:10, Amplified)

My assignment is to accept it *gladly* even if I have to go through major surgery, then radiology, chemo or whatever. If there is no way but through, the Lord will put a *tent over me.* He will shelter me through the fire, flood, valley, trauma, pain, weakness and all the "whatevers" that may caboose my days while I'm in my mortal, failing body.

Heavenly helicopter

I have never gone mountain climbing. Nor have I ever climbed an illness mountain like this one. I've watched others, *but now it's my turn.* I feel as if I'm climbing it all alone without anyone holding the rope above me.

But I know better. The Lord has shown me in these days of preparation that not only is *He* with me, but I have a host of *friends* firmly holding the ropes by prayer. This surgical adventure is not just a foothill to me. It's a "biggie," like Mt. Everest. What's more, I don't know if this is my final mountain or the first of many mountains in the same range.

As the gospel song declares, "I've come this far by faith, leaning on the Lord." Surely He will prove as strong and faithful on my behalf as He has before. It is God who holds the rope. He is ahead of me and above me. His strong grip will not let me fall. The top of this mountain may be the best lookout view of life God has ever given me, although the climb may be the most difficult. If I slip down the other side of this mountain into a valley, I'm sure to find the greenest grass and freshest water there.

We can't have mountains without valleys between. The Lord of the Valley invites me to go with Him through the valley and promises that I shall not want. How dull and monotonous if life were nothing but flat prairies!

When I arrive at tomorrow's mountain, I'm counting on the Lord's tender compassion and love. He promised not to give me more than I can bear. I'll set my heart on "things above" and count on God to take care of all my mountain climbing arrangements.

Maybe He'll provide a spiritual cable car. Perhaps a *heavenly helicopter* (my guardian angel?) to lift me up and carry me over. I'll be airborne on His mighty wings swooping over that mountain. From God's heights, I'll look down on my mountain and it will seem no more formidable than foothills. The words of another song keep coming to me:

> Things over my head, are under His feet;
> Things I can't begin, He can complete;
> There's a mountain ahead that I can't climb,
> But God can carry me over.

God's promise from Isaiah 43:2,3 is reassurance from His Control Tower:

> When you pass through the waters, I will be with you; and through the rivers, they will not overflow you. When you walk through the fire, you will not be scorched, nor will the flame burn you. For I am the Lord your God, the Holy One. . . . ◆

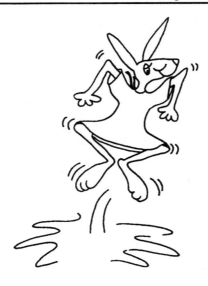

My Personal Workout

1. What are my fears and anxieties about my illness at this point?

2. What actual physical symptoms can fear cause? Do I experience any?

3. In what practical way could I cast specific fears on the Lord?

4. How does Philippians 4:6,7 work for me right now?

5. What verses might I memorize which would be meaningful in my time of need?

6. Am I trying to make any deal with God to get me through this situation?

7. What attitude could I have that would please God more?

Part 2

Mid-Op: This is IT! Submerged

Paging the reader . . . paging the reader . . .

If you want to stay in the WAITING ROOM while I'm in surgery, you may skip this section. God willing, I'll see you in my hospital room when I'm back from ICU in Part Three.

However, I hope you'll stay with me through this section. Look at it either as a dry run for your (or someone's) future hospital adventure or a comparison with your unique experience.

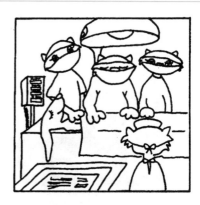

Chapter 7

Are We Having Fun Yet?

P re-admittance hospital instructions read: "Eat a nourishing supper and a snack before bedtime. Take a bath or shower, wash your hair, and remove any nail polish. Then nothing by mouth after midnight. This means no food or even coffee, juice, water or chewing gum. Your stomach must be as empty as possible before your surgery to prevent complications from anesthesia."

The time has come. It's the night before (not Christmas, that's for sure!) surgery, and all through the house not a creature is stirring . . . I hope not a mouse. It's dreadfully quiet and routine. I'm still at home. My family is asleep. I'm not sure I agree with the policy of same day admittance for surgery. This is the night before my "mountain climb," and I feel completely alone.

I drink three glasses of water at exactly one minute before midnight, although I don't usually drink water at night. I feel so deprived already. My bedside digital clock blinks its silent red eyes while its numbers drag their feet toward dawn.

I need rest, but sleep eludes me. My mouth is already dry as the Saudi desert. How long before I'll drink water again? Can I survive without it? I'm not a camel.

My courage is slowly leaking away. I'm not leaning into the wind. It's my last chance to have a business meeting with God before dawn.

Meeting called to order: I don't have time to read the Minutes of all my struggles of the last few weeks. Time is running out. *Lord, search my heart for any old business or new business on Your agenda.*

What seems to bother me most about this surgical adventure and my illness is that *I'm not in control.* I'm used to being self-sufficient, independent and able to cope. My attitude may sometimes have been: *I can do it, plan it, control it (and almost bless it) myself.* I fall too easily into the world's pattern of the go-getter, the doer, the goal-setter, the high achiever. My attitude may have been: "I have it within me, in my will power and my ability to accomplish what I believe God has called me to do."

I'm looking into a mirror now. Is it *humility* that I lack?

Is that one major lesson You're trying to teach me? Lord, I want to move toward Christian maturity. That may mean that I should become less independent and more dependent upon You. That's the opposite of human maturity where the goal is independence. I must realize that what I am and what I do is truly not under my control. Is my illness a tutor whom You've sent to instruct me toward humility and maturity?

I know I can't drive the vehicle of my life properly by my own wisdom. In the first place, the vehicle isn't mine, it's Yours. The fuel, too, must come from Your pump. The best I can put into my tank is the cheapest grade. Yours is super-premium, high-test fuel. It's You, Lord, who gives me the "Trip Tick" map for my life. You highlight the roads I'm to take and detours I should make. You ordain the length of my life journey.

I know this isn't really new business. I have already surrendered to You, God. Your will has been my sincere lifetime desire. Yet to embrace this deeper humility is something essential that I can learn only from a life-threatening illness, surgery or accident over which I have no control.

Lord, humility hasn't been high on my list of "most wanted" character traits. But apparently You consider it indispensable if I want to be conformed to the image of Christ. Then have Your own way, Lord. "Look! No hands!" I bow my head willingly and lean forward toward whatever You have prepared for me in the morning.

Business meeting adjourned.

Brief and restless sleep takes over.

Strangely dim

I'm in the hospital. The time has finally come.

Some concerns instantly leap into bold relief, and other things "grow strangely dim," as the hymn writer expressed it. Surgery forces me to "turn my eyes upon Jesus, look full in His wonderful face." Perhaps I might look at His face a lot sooner than I expected.

A perky, young, medical attendant in a white uniform fastens a plastic I.D. bracelet on my wrist. Then she smiles and thrusts a clipboard at me with a long list of possible complications during my forthcoming surgery. "Go over them carefully, and I'll be back in a few minutes." She pulls the curtain across the door of my little undressing cubicle and disappears.

I scan the list with growing apprehension. Perspiration begins to dampen my brow. What a catalog of possibilities, eventualities, dangers and "worst case" risks ahead of me! The hospital wants me to be aware that I might have cardiac arrest, hemorrhage to death, my lungs might collapse, certain procedures may cause paralysis of some part of me, doctors might discover that a malignancy has spread beyond hope . . . there are more . . . .

The young lady returns and cheerfully explains some surgery terminology and procedures, then asks if I understand. *Yes, I guess I understand.* Suddenly, I'm like the little child clutching a Teddy bear in the TV commercial that promotes new CAT scan procedures. I feel like whimpering, "Mommy, I wanna go home!" Fear ties my stomach in knots. My face feels flushed. My hands tremble. I haven't eaten since yesterday, but that's not my problem. The three monsters (panic, anxiety and fear) that I thought I conquered have returned to attack me with renewed vigor.

There is no way but through. She hands me a ballpoint pen and shows me where to sign to indicate that I understand and consent to the proposed surgical procedure "and whatever else related to it might become necessary."

I've reached a point of no return. I sign.

Eternity comes into focus. Daily concerns of a transient nature that were so important yesterday blur into insignificance. They are passing incidentals, temporal, of this earth, tied to time. I may have run out of time. The spotlight is focused on my relationship with God. Little else matters. Time seemed to stretch endlessly when everything was going smoothly in the past. Now I can't even count on tomorrow.

Have I come only to a *comma* in my life, a slight pause, or to a period, a *full stop*? Only God knows. Maybe I've reached the end of the sentence, the paragraph, the chapter—the book?

I have faith in God that if I don't come through this surgical adventure, I'll find myself immediately in His presence. I've settled all that. But I secretly hope to stick around planet Earth a little longer. *Thinking positive thoughts doesn't seem to help me, Lord. Let me hear from you directly.* "I say to you, do not be anxious for your life . . . therefore do not be anxious for tomorrow; for tomorrow will take care for itself. Each day has enough trouble of its own" (Matthew 6:25, 34).

That's for sure, Lord. But it is today I'm anxious about—the next few hours. Please give me a double dose of Your peace. Calm my raging, inward storm with Your "Peace! Be still!"

You promised never to leave me or forsake me. I grasp for Your presence, Lord. "Lo, I am with you always, even to the end of the age" (Matthew 28:20). To the end of this planet? To the end of my life in old age? To the end of my earthly life now? *All of the above, please.* I focus on the assurance that looking "full in His wonderful face" is not worst case—it is the best case!

All right, let earth grow dim and heaven be illuminated!

The waiting game

"You must be at the hospital before seven a.m." they instructed me. Fine. A long predawn drive got us here on schedule. Paperwork took a half hour, final instructions and change into hospital gown and other details took another half hour.

Then I went to "The Parking Lot" on the surgical floor where a horrendous hold up began. A veritable traffic jam. Why did I agree to be surgical patient #2 this morning? I should have insisted on being the first, even if I had to get up at three a.m. to get to the hospital. This practice of same day admittance and surgery has turned out to be a bummer.

I've been waiting more than five hours, prepped and impatient! In my breezy hospital gown, in a wheel-chair, covered with blankets, in the surgical lounge which is like Grand Central Station. They parked me in front of a television set, gave me magazines, told me that I may still have *a few hours to wait!* Nothing by mouth *for me,* of course, but the nursing staff laughs, drinks cokes, munches nachos, and my husband went down to the cafeteria for coffee and a donut!

I loathe being in limbo like this. I have an impatient temperament.. The anticipation, suspense and uncertainty are almost more than I can bear. I thought my mind and emotions were well-anchored to faith, trust and all those courageous thoughts I counted on. Now cold, clammy fear grips me by the shoulder. Am I expected to spend what may be my final hours of life watching a stupid game show or sit-com? I would have been a lot braver if they had let me march in quickly, lie down, have the anesthesia and get on with it.

A thoughtful nurse comes to assure me that my long wait is because of the unexpected length of the previous patient's surgery. "Probably some unforeseen complications," she remarks. That's no comfort. I already know that *his* scheduled surgery was the *same as mine!* I am edgy.

"I've been informed," says the nurse, "that due to your long wait you'll skip 'The Holding Area.' *(I thought that's where I was!)* You'll be wheeled directly from here to O.R." That's a relief!

Ten o'clock—eleven o'clock—twelve o'clock— one o'clock. My husband goes out for lunch. And returns. We kiss and say goodbye *again.*

But I *didn't* escape "The Holding Area" after all! They wheeled me out of the fancy lounge and *parked me again* in a curtained-off area at an unidentified location. Then they left me alone. No one else is in this new parking lot. I'm shivering with only a thin blanket over my hospital gown. Every time a door opens somewhere I feel a draft. There's no "call button" on my gurney to summon someone. I feel like unstrapping myself from the gurney and running like the wind out of here!

I'm all alone. The big, round clock on the wall in front of me with its white stoic face and black hands is the only thing keeping an eye on me. Ten minutes, twenty, thirty, forty minutes—Did they forget me? Why no ticket for overtime parking?

The joking of doctors and nurses somewhere beyond the curtain, laughter, the clink-clank of routine sounds float around me. That irritates me because I'm sedated only enough to be fuzzy, but not enough to doze off or sleep through the delay.

Plenty of action on the other side of the curtain, however. The smell of fresh-brewed coffee makes my empty stomach growl. I hear surgeons dictating post-operative reports into tape recorders. Drowsy and groggy, I can only turn my numb-dumb head far enough to peep through the small gap between two curtains.

I see a post-op patient on a gurney with IV lines and tubes attached to him. Several nurses keep calling his name. "Brian, Brian. Wake up. Your surgery is over. Can you open your eyes? Wake up now."

Lucky him! But *I'm* not done yet. I'm not even *begun!* When will they come for me? I don't want to be here alone. My husband wasn't allowed to come into this area. I'm strapped and helpless on this cold gurney in some forsaken area.

God, where are You? Have You forsaken me? I've lost Your promised presence. I can't even pray. Where are those sustaining Bible verses? I must have left my courage in the bag with my street clothes. This awful limbo! I've been in this new parking lot another whole, long hour!

Prayer from the gurney

Lord, aloneness is swallowing me up. The chilly feeling deep in the pit of my stomach is taking over my whole body. I feel like they've shoved me into a dank, dark cave where I'm all alone. Yes, I'm afraid!

You know I'm a first-timer in this hospital experience. The childbirth experiences don't really count. They were happy events to which I looked forward. I've never walked in such emotional darkness before, and the eyes of my heart aren't accustomed to it. I can't see, hear, or feel anyone else around. It's as if I don't have a light to see my surroundings.

If only I could reach out and touch someone— anyone. I need to know that another person has grappled with the same fear, struggled with the same questions.

"I am the light of the world," Jesus said. "He who follows Me shall not walk in the darkness, but shall have the light of life" (John 8:12), "Lo, I am with you always. . . ." (Matthew 28:20).

Whether I feel Him or not, Jesus is here and I have His light! I can see that I'm not in a cave but in a tunnel. A cave has only one entrance; it's confining and claustrophobic. But my tunnel not only has an entrance, it has an exit! Not only is there a light at the end of the tunnel, but God's Great Light floods the whole tunnel.

When I get through this incredible adventure, Lord, I will be a debtor. When You bring me out of this tunnel, I want to walk other newcomers through. I want to reach out and squeeze their hands and let them know they aren't alone. You understand their fears. And now I do too. You will walk through dark times together with us.

Even though I walk through the valley of the shadow of death, I fear no evil; for Thou art with me. (Psalm 23:4)

Blessed be the God and Father of our Lord Jesus Christ, the Father of mercies and

God of all comfort, who comforts us in all our
affliction so that we may be able to comfort
those who are in any affliction with the comfort
with which we ourselves are comforted by God.
(2 Corinthians 1:3,4)

Bulldog grip

Finally they are pushing me toward the operating
room! *Now is the time* to recall some of those promises
from God that I've practiced, recorded on tape and
memorized.

Whoa—I can't get my thoughts in gear! My mind
is stuck in woolly neutral. It doesn't function. They've
just given me new medication and it's taking effect. I've
become mentally shallow and muddled. My mind sloshes
around randomly grasping for what it should know—but
doesn't. Reality fades.

Not even *one* Bible verse floats within reach for my
mind to grasp. I struggle to concentrate, but my thoughts
are a flat line. I reach for God. I must find Him in this misty
maze of my need. *Where are You, Lord?* "We have
waited for Thee eagerly; Thy name, even Thy memory,
is the desire of our souls. Indeed, my spirit within me
seeks Thee diligently" (Isaiah 8:9).

When a Bible verse floats by, I grab for it, try to bite
into it and hold on like a bulldog sinking its teeth into the
seat of an intruder's pants. At last I have one! "Thou wilt
keep him in perfect peace. . . ." That's only part of it. I
can't remember the rest or its Bible address while I'm in
this twilight zone, although I know it well.

Anyway, who cares?
I chew this short, bite-size promise from God over and over like gum. I keep repeating it. Only one thought takes up the entire space in my blurred brain which seems to have shrunk in capacity.

"Thou wilt keep him in perfect peace . . . in perfect peace . . ." I repeat the words to the slow rhythm of my breathing. In and out, in and out: "in perfect peace. . . ."

At first I'm able to whisper the words. Then I can only lip-sink them to mesh with my thoughts. No sound comes out, but the truth lingers. It is in my spirit, in my mind. Brightly emblazoned on my brain. The promised peace of God seeps into my inner spirit like a vapor or mist. *My whole being is permeated with God's peace.*

At last I must be nearly sedated, but my spirit and breathing pattern are still slowly pumping into me that precious, life-giving promise and appropriating God's peace. I relax. God is in control. *I'm flying on automatic pilot now,* in His capable hands. "In perfect peace . . . in perfect peace. . . ."

Absolute surrender

I vaguely remember the brilliance of the overhead lights in the O.R. illuminating my motionless body strapped and clamped to the cold surgical table. The Preparatory Booklet said I might be aware of a clean smell, soft music, and people talking. *Wait a minute! That could also describe heaven!*

The medication in my veins floats me into total unconsciousness. For a fleeting moment I realize just how complete is my relinquishment to the procedures and the people who hold my life in their hands. I have trusted them totally. Sounds recede. Faces blur then disappear. I've slipped into neutral darkness where I have no dreams, no visions. I am suspended in nothingness without feelings. I'm unaware of what is being done to my human body.

My life is committed to the hands of my chief surgeon and his team, at the mercy of their education, skill, experience, alertness, judgment. And perhaps affected by what they had for breakfast, and whether or not they are getting along with their spouses or significant others. They are only human beings like me, mortals who, although highly competent, are fallible!

I wouldn't trust them if I were not sure that I had angelic "security guards" who answer to the Great Physician. When the president of the United States appears in public, I've watched the plain clothes guards around him. They stand quietly, but they observe everything going on. Their experienced eyes dart to and fro watching for anything out of the ordinary.

I'm counting on my angelic security guards to keep their eyes on those white-clad operators who were arguing about last night's football game as they scrubbed up.

Now I understand more fully what complete surrender means. God invites me, instructs me, beseeches me by His mercies and love to surrender myself, my life, my all to him. That is total submission, not unlike my experience as I lie on the operating table. "I urge you therefore, brethren, by the mercies of God, to present your bodies a living and holy sacrifice, acceptable to God, which is your spiritual service of worship" (Romans 12:1).

Why would I not surrender completely to such a loving God and trust Him with my mortal life and my immortal spirit? I belong to an infallible, almighty, all-knowing, totally loving, all-wise Master. He holds the keys to life and death, heaven and hell. As my Creator, He holds my life-breath in His hands.

The procedure God wants to do in my life is spiritual surgery. He can cut out my malignancy of sin, restore me whole, transfuse me with His blood and re-create me in His image. Then He strengthens me by His own Spirit to walk recovered before Him in newness of life. His work is not only in my spirit, but in my body.

I've prayed, and so have my friends, that my surgeon will be the proxy hands of God, an instrument to accomplish God's purpose for me. How thankful I am that he, too, is a child of God, a praying man.

A Surgeon's Prayer

Dear God:
These strong gloved fingers
which I flex—
this human hand
which holds the knife,
sterile now and steady,
needs Thy guiding skill
to help another life.

Bless now this patient—
Thine and mine—
who, under Thee, entrusts to me
a precious life!

God of the surgeon's tireless strength,
the surgeon's finite skill,
grant that I may guided be
to do Thy will.
Amen.

(Author Unknown)

Ticket to an operating theater

They call the O.R. an "Operating Theater" for good reason! Everyone gathers around to see the main attraction. *Me!* The place is like an amphitheater, an arena, a stage. I'm exposed, displayed, on exhibit. It's a good thing I'm totally *"out to lunch."* I would be so embarrassed. I'm thankful that I have no idea what's going on. I must appear most undignified lying here.

I'm only partially covered. I do wear an unfashionable surgical "designer" cap. *But I also wear a crown!* In fact, it's a *double* crown. "He crowns you with *lovingkindness and compassion"* (Psalm 103:4). Other translations say that "to crown" means "to beautify, dignify." I'm sure I need that! "Lovingkindness" is steadfast love, unfailing love, God's love. "Compassion" is also translated as tender mercies.

Thank you. I'll take a heaping portion of both of the above from the generous hand of my loving Lord God!

The surgical team, the medical technicians, the whole "crowd of witnesses" that "encompass me round about" won't see any crowns, but I claim them. Since God provided them, they are visible to Him. "O continue Thy lovingkindness to those who know Thee, and Thy righteousness to the upright in heart" (Psalm 36:10).

I do know You, Lord, and my righteousness is drawn only from the righteousness of Jesus. I'm not upright in body because I'm horizontal on the O.R. table. But my heart is upright toward You. Lord, You say that Your lovingkindness extends to the heavens. I ask that it may cover me down here in the O.R. in my hour of need.

Yes, Lord, please continue Your lovingkindness: prolong it, stretch it out, keep it going, lengthen it. I need both Your intensive care in this emergency and Your extended care for the long haul of my recovery—if I make it through.

My God-given crowns may become a little lop-sided during the long hours of surgery, but of one thing I'm sure: God will see to it that my crowns don't fall off!

Wake up call

After an unknown period of time, I drift toward consciousness aware that someone is calling a name and squeezing my hand. I don't answer. I can't. Besides, I don't know if it's *my* name. I'm not sure *who* I am. I feel exposed, vulnerable. I seem to be the center of attention. So many people hover around me and hurry back and forth. In the background I'm aware of a high-pitched, steady beeping.

I sneak a peek with unfocused eyes through droopy eyelids. "They" are in white! Does the fluttering noise come from wings? Are they angels? Did I finish my race on earth and enter my immortal existence? My thoughts are fuzzy. I can't grasp reality. It takes too much effort to think. I drift in and out of a twilight zone. I'm tired, oh, so tired.

"They" persist in calling a name. It's beginning to sound a bit familiar. Some are engaging in small talk, laughing. Someone says, "As soon as she comes out of it, let's go for coffee and Danish." Another remarks, "Say, did you get a load of that new hunk of an intern?" *I doubt this is heaven!*

Somewhere else in the room "they" are calling another name. Is *that* me? Or is *this* body me?

Involuntarily, I move slightly. Ouch! This body hurts! So I can't be immortal yet. Oh, how it hurts! Let me sleep. Please!

No luck. "They" keep hassling me into consciousness. Finally I try to reply, but a breathing tube fills my mouth and throat. I can't swallow. I can't reply! I'm not in control of my movements. I'm at the mercy of whatever is happening to me.

Finally, to oblige "them," I try to blink my eyes, the only part of me that I can move without hurting. I grunt. I moan. I roll my head. Finally they are satisfied!

"Good girl, good girl!" someone croons, patting my arm. *That's what I say to my dog!*

"Your surgery is over now," someone whispers. Well, I sure hope so! *Thank You, Lord, thank You, Lord!*

Oh, just let me sleep, let me sleep again. It even hurts to think. Pain—oh, it would be better if "they" *were* angels and this *was* heaven. I'd fly, yes, I'd fly . . . and I wouldn't hurt. . . .

In ICU

I drift in and out of consciousness innumerable times. Where did I decide I was? Earth or heaven? I forgot my conclusion. I only know that I hurt. I can't move. So it's *not* heaven. Must be the Intensive Care Unit.

I lie connected to life support systems and tubes in nearly every orifice. A drainage tube from my side, a tube down my throat leading to a respirator, a suction tube hanging from the corner of my mouth to rid me of phlegm. I have round patches stuck to my chest wired to a heart monitor. IV lines drip medications into my veins, and a blood pressure cuff is around my arm. I'm attached to a catheter and a PCA button dispensing pain medicine is taped to my wrist and connected to apparatus beside my bed.

A gadget is taped to my fingertip with a red light on it. I feel like E.T., the Extra-Terrestrial in the movie, who pleaded, "E.T. wants to go home!" So do I!

With a breathing tube down my throat, I can't communicate. That sensation is worse than the pain. I think I'm going to have a panic attack. I feel claustrophobic.

I need help! Where's my call button? My hand doesn't respond to my brain. The button dangles beyond my reach over the bars at my bedside. *Help! I'm gagging on the breathing tube!* My throat is constricting and I can't swallow. What if I survived surgery but died of suffocation? I can't tell anyone what's wrong!

No nurses are around me at the moment. They're all busy attending to other patients in what seems to be a large, very crowded room. Only pull-around curtains separate patients. I have no way to get attention. I break out in cold sweat.

Finally someone comes. I try to mumble. I gag.

My mouth is so dry. I'm desperate to find out how long I must have this wretched breathing tube down my throat. How can I make myself understood? I try to point to my breathing tube and shake my head. "Don't move now, dearie. We'll remove the tube in about 24 hours."

Great! They can read my mind!

Twenty-four hours! I don't even know what day it is or how long since my surgery. My family isn't here. Do I have a family? Where are they? What time of the day or night is it?

I continue to try to communicate. The frustrated nurse leaves and then returns with a clipboard and pencil murmuring, "Write it down, dearie." She puts a pencil in my taped-down hand, and it falls right out again. Is she kidding? What does she expect of a post-op patient? Finally I think I made some scratches on the paper, but I have no idea what they are or even what I want to write. My mind stalls. I don't have strength to turn the ignition key again. She brings a cool, wet cloth for my forehead. Bless her!

If only I could have some water! How long since I've had water? Before midnight days ago, it seems. I try to write the word "water" on the clipboard. No luck. With my strapped-down hand, I try to point to my mouth. "I'll bring you a little piece of ice, dearie." Ah, good guess! I savor the ice as if it were the choicest morsel in the world. But I keep gagging when I try to swallow because of the breathing tube.

She leaves for a while, and tells me to hold the suction device myself. *Impossible!* I'm too sedated to hold on to it. It falls to the pillow, and I can't retrieve it.

On the other side of the separating curtain I can hear a whole group of people talking to someone they're calling Ed. Are people supposed to have so many visitors in ICU? Their murmuring and whispers drift in and out of my ultra-sensitive ears and confuse me. Why are they here in the middle of the night? Or is it daytime? They never turn the lights off. The entire ICU is so brightly illuminated it's impossible to tell whether it's day or night.

Nurses have been calling the name "Brian" over and over somewhere in ICU behind another curtain where I hear someone thrashing violently on the bed. Suddenly silence. Where there was an intermittent beeping sound, it has now flat-lined. They stop calling that name. Before long the curtains are drawn back, and I'm aware that a silent form is being wheeled out. An orderly stands ready to push a freshly-made bed to the vacated spot.

Plain pain

The pre-admittance instruction booklet I received at my first hospital appointment explained "After Surgery Procedures."

"Pain medication is available after surgery. Ask for it when you need it. Please do not wait until you can no longer tolerate your pain because medication takes time to begin working. Incisional pain is often described as 'aching,' 'sharp,' or 'pulling.'"

Tell me about it! All the above and "other!" This post-op pain is my first encounter with intense pain, since I don't count my four childbirth experiences. After those, you have something wonderful to show for your pain and you forget it. Now I have a remarkable electronic pain medication dispenser called a PCA.

The nurse reminds me that I shouldn't try to be

brave but push the PCA button as often as I need it. She says I can't overdose because the portion is pre-measured, and the device is timed. Time means nothing to me in this zombie state. I think I must be pushing the button all the time and keeping myself sedated, trying to hurry the time until I can get out of ICU. I have no problem with trying to be brave. I'm cowardly!

Pain. A strange experience. An unwanted one. But if it takes pain to heal my problem, I'll endure it. The Bible talks about "momentary light affliction" (2 Corinthians 4:17). I don't think the apostle Paul was referring to the pain of surgery and illness, but I guess it could still apply. It doesn't seem momentary to me, nor light. In perspective, I guess it is. Pain is for this life only.

The apostle Paul said it was productive. "Producing for us an eternal weight of glory far beyond all comparison." I repeat in my fuzzy mind, "momentary light affliction . . . momentary light affliction . . . ." I doze off under the medication.

I come back to consciousness by hearing someone groan. *It's me!* I make strange noises because of that thick breathing tube. I'm not groaning with complaint, but involuntarily, with a kind of basic, earthy quality common to human pain.

"Indeed, in this house we groan" (2 Corinthians 5:2,4). In this house, my human body, my earthly tent. So fragile, so easily torn, so subject to high winds and storms, age deterioration, made with hands, mortal, subject to infirmity.

My mind, only partly under my control, begins to toy with the idea of trading in the pain and groaning of my earthly tent for the substantial "building" Scripture talks about—the dwelling from heaven, not made with hands, immortal, eternal in the heavens, swallowed up by life, not death.

The nurse has pulled aside my curtain, and now I can see the big, round wall clock. Both hands point to two. Afternoon? In the middle of the night?

I punch the PCA again. And again. I drift off. I can think of only one word: *Jesus.* I repeat it in my spirit over and over. *Jesus. Jesus. Jesus.* The two syllables coincide with my breath inhaled, exhaled. I sink my anchor on *the name of Jesus* and let Him hold me. I could never hang on to life by myself. My grasp is too weak. *Jesus, tie Your rope safely around me as I bob in the water drifting to and fro, in and out of consciousness.*

Hold me, keep me, help me endure. Let the time pass. Let morning come soon, come soon, come soon . . . "My soul waits for the Lord more than the watchmen for the morning; indeed, more than the watchmen for the morning" (Psalm 130:6).

Comes with the package

Before my surgery I never gave much thought to breathing. I took it for granted. It came with the package of my body machinery activated at birth. Given by the Lord, of course.

After they removed the breathing tube that pumped just the right amount of air from the respirator into my repaired lungs, I can still not breathe on my own. I use an oxygen mask strapped to my face which keeps slipping off. But thank God we're making progress.

I had plenty of time during my extended hospital stay to think about the awesome spiritual significance of breath and breathing. It is unique to God's created ones.

In Genesis 2:7 it is recorded that God breathed into the nostrils of the first man, and he became a living soul. *God breathes,* whatever that really means. We receive our breath from Him.

When the frightened disciples gathered after His resurrection, Jesus "breathed on them and said to them, 'Receive the Holy Spirit'" (John 20:22). With the first breathing into us we began life. With the second breathing we received "life more abundantly" (John 10:10). "Life in all its fullness," as the Living Bible paraphrased it.

How completely dependent I am upon God for life through breathing! My brain can't function without oxygen inhaled through breathing. And when my breath stops, my earthly life comes to a halt.

It seems inconceivable but they say that in a 24-hour period an adult breathes about 23,040 times. What a ventilating system, what an air-conditioner our Creator has installed in our bodies! How marvelous that God designed two lungs, not identical, with their five lobes which take in the perfect mixture of air that He provided in Earth's atmosphere! I use about 438 cubic feet of that air daily and automatically! That would fill some huge balloon!

Literally, my breath, my life, is in the hands of the Lord. It's up to Him to stop my breathing or to keep it going. In Daniel 5:23 I'm reminded how important it is to give credit and honor to God who gives me breath. "God *in whose hand is your breath,* and whose are all your ways, you have not honored."

After this surgical adventure, I'll never take breathing for granted again. The Living Bible paraphrases Acts 17:25, "He Himself gives life and breath to everything, and satisfies every need there is."

How shall I express appreciation to my Lord for this marvelous apparatus of lungs and related body parts of nose and mouth designed to automatically take in the air allowing me to continue living? David has the golden words again, "Let everything that hath breath praise the Lord. Praise *ye* the Lord!" (Psalm 150:6)

I do, Lord, I sure do! Praise You, thank You, Lord! ◆

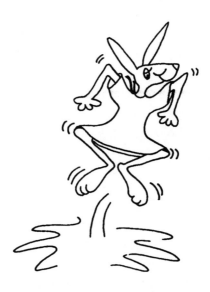

My Personal Workout

1. If I have had (or am having) a hospital adventure, have I prayed for my doctors, surgeon and all the hospital staff attending me?

2. How did my own experience in surgery compare with the author's?

3. In what specific ways did God help me deal with fear, anxiety, pain and discomfort?

4. How have I expressed my thanks to God for sustaining me through times of physical distress?

Part 3

Post-Op: Emerging

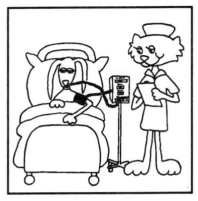

Chapter 8

Working My Way Through Spiritual College

*L*ord, help me remember that nothing is going to happen to me today that you and I together can't handle.

A friend stuck a little card with the above affirmation on it into one of my get-well cards. I sink my teeth firmly into that morsel of God's truth.

After three days, I'm finally out of ICU. Praise God! All things pass! I'm still connected to most of the wires and tubes, but I'm carefully breathing on my own now. Orderlies came to transfer me from ICU to a regular room. They are settling me in and adjusting my sundry attachments. Another patient, a pre-op, is being moved into the second bed. Nurses leave me alone for a minute while they attend to her behind the drawn curtain.

Suddenly I feel as if my bed is shaking. Is it an earthquake? I put my hands on my chest. The pounding and shaking are *inside me!* My heart beats become wild and erratic, fluttering and jumping around. Blood is pounding in my ears and behind my ears. *Scary!* My heart races, stops, leaps, slows, then races again!

I clench my call button. "Something's wrong with me! Help!" A nurse runs to my bedside, briefly feels my pulse, then whips out her blood pressure cuff while pressing an emergency call button. More nurses run into my room. The head nurse barks, "Call the floor resident, STAT!" He arrives in a few seconds on the run and targets me with his stethoscope even before reaching my bed.

Nurses constantly monitor my pulse and blood pressure. The doctor quickly orders medication injected into my vein, one dose after another. Then medication is added to my IV line. They wire me to a device which produces a graph on a long tape which several attendants study intently. *Lord, help me remember that nothing is going to happen to me today that you and I together can't handle.*

I lie quietly, strangely at peace, somehow detached, floating, as if what is going on is happening to someone else. "The Lord is a very present help in time of trouble" (Psalm 46:1). *Did I survive surgery only to die of a heart attack? O.K., if that's what You want, Lord. I guess.*

Within an hour, everything settles down, but

nurses don't leave me alone for a minute. The blood pressure cuff stays on my arm. The head nurse informs me they are transferring me to a single room next door, Room 12, where a heart monitor is permanently installed in the wall.

For the next four days, I stay wired to it by plastic suction cups attached to my chest. They unhook me temporarily when I sit in a chair or walk to the bathroom. Every two hours day and night they wake me for blood pressure, pulse and temperature readings.

My pulse and heart rate are digitally displayed on the monitor behind my bed. A graph constantly prints out my heart rhythm, and doctors study it daily before they post it on my bulletin board. Later my doctor told me that about 30 percent of post-operative patients who have had heart or lung surgery experience such an arrhythmic spasm.

You and I handled it, Lord, didn't we? Blessed be the name of the Lord. My heart is in Your hands, literally, moment by moment, heart beat by heart beat.

All that is within me

I've become intensely conscious of what is happening inside me in this surgical classroom because doctors and nurses monitor me constantly. I memorized the first few verses of Psalm 103 for such a time as this. "Bless the Lord, O my soul; and *all that is within me*, bless His holy name."

All that is within me? All my internal organs which God created, yes. How about all those tubes, wires and connections within me? The internal stitches, the scars, the metal clips, the resections? Apparently so. I am to bless God's holy name *with my soul,* which is unseen, unmonitored. It is the only part of me that is free and under my control. My eternal spirit is not shackled.

I am not in any church building. Nevertheless, I can bless the Lord, I can praise the Lord, I can worship the Lord. "Bless the Lord, O my soul, and forget none of His benefits" (103:2). I lie here counting them. Not one by one, but ton by ton!

"Who pardons all your iniquities" (103:3). Thank God. I lie here redeemed by faith in the blood of Jesus Christ offered on Calvary for my salvation. If life-support systems fail, or my body ceases to heal and respond, I know I'll immediately enter the presence of God clothed in His righteousness and live with Him eternally. I thank God for sins no longer *within me.*

"Who heals all your diseases" (103:3). Thank God. There is nothing too hard for Him, no matter what my physical condition. Surgeons have limitations. The Great Physician doesn't. I bless the Lord for the skill of surgeons and caregivers, sterile facilities, medications and life-support systems aiding my battered body to recover. Bless God for built-in restorative powers that God put *within me.* Bless the Lord for His healing power at work even beyond the natural.

"Who redeems your life from the pit (from destruction)" (103:4). I thank the Lord that I came through surgery, that I still have life *within me.*

"Who crowns you with lovingkindness and compassion" (103:4). A generation ago, even less, medical science had not advanced to the point of the present surgical skill and care that I am receiving.

"Who satisfies your years with good things, so that your youth is renewed like the eagle" (103:5). I ask the

Lord, if He wills, that He might renew my life and extend it for some years because of the procedures done on me. Perhaps I may have another chance at life and joy, and a longer time to glorify the Lord through carrying out His purposes in me. Length of years or not, *I have this day.* One day at a time.

"Bless the Lord, all you works of His." *That's me, Lord. I am Your workmanship, created in Christ Jesus.* (Ephesians 2:10) "In all places of His dominion." *Yes, even in this hospital bed. I claim Room 12 as Your territory, Your dominion! "Bless the Lord, O my soul!"* (103:22).

My light affliction

What do I really know about pain? I push a button to dispense medication which alleviates my pain. Nurses give me pills to dull it. I lie in antiseptic privacy in the hush of Room 12. My thoughts drift to Jesus Christ. What do I really know about "the fellowship of His sufferings? My surgery saved me from death. They deliberately put Jesus to death.

The pain Jesus suffered on the cross is unparalleled torture of the worst kind. It is SUFFERING in capital letters. Soldiers inflicted pain to deliberately abuse Him, to cause Him the most excruciating agony. His tormenters laughed with hellish pleasure to see Him writhe in anguish.

Anesthesia did not relieve His pain.

They crucified Jesus in the most public place possible, along a dusty, traveled road and near a market. They stripped him in full view of the unsympathetic, mocking crowd and before those who loved Him. Some

unrealistic artists who let their imaginations run wild have
painted crucifixion scenes on a lovely, grassy hill. Movie
makers added background music. No such thing. His
was a criminal's death. More like an angry mob lynch-
ing. The authorities meant to make it a public example,
to strike fear and disgust in the hearts of His followers and
bystanders. Hecklers were said to hope that a criminal's
agony would be prolonged and they would jeer loudly to
arouse the emotions of the victim.

By contrast my room is quiet and private. The
hospital staff is solicitous. They attend to my every ache
or pain or need and continually monitor my vital signs.
I was tenderly prepped for surgery and fortified with IVs
for my sterile ordeal.

But Jesus was beaten, scourged and spit on. His
head must have throbbed fiercely from the crown of
thorns brutal men fiendishly shoved down upon His
forehead. His face was bloody, bruised and disfigured
from their savage blows. Weakened, He was paraded to
drag a splintery, massive wooden cross along a public
thoroughfare before the townspeople. His back was raw
and mutilated. Depraved men viciously pounded huge
rusty nails into Jesus' hands and feet, piercing through
flesh and bone.

They only pierced my delicate flesh gently with a
sterile needle to dull my senses and render me peacefully
unconscious while careful, skillful surgeons made pur-
poseful cuts in my body. They intended such incisions
for my healing not for the sadistic pleasure of men with
twisted minds. They quickly replenished my loss of
blood, but blood hemorrhaged from Jesus' body
unchecked, spilling on the ground beneath the cross.

My brief suffering, even at its worst, is not worthy

to compare with His. I dare not say I even faintly experienced "the fellowship of His sufferings." I tiptoe on the fringes of understanding what pain is all about, although it is greater than I ever experienced. My small taste of discomfort makes me cherish and esteem the precious suffering of Christ in a solemn, fresh way.

Nevertheless, the suffering of Jesus Christ was not an end in itself. He suffered *for me!* Jesus redeemed my soul through His affliction and death. He didn't suffer for His own wrongdoing, but for the sins of all humankind laid on Him during His ordeal on the cross. He drank the cup of pain to the last drop to atone for mankind's sin— for mine. The Father must have lifted the veil to let Him see into the future, to understand that His suffering provided eternal salvation for whoever would accept His work on Calvary.

And I *do. I do!* I accept His suffering for me, *for me!* My heart is overwhelmed with gratitude for His redemptive accomplishment for me.

"The Big C"

Do I have a major or minor illness? Sometimes we draw a distinction between a heart attack, stroke and "The Big C" (cancer) on one side . . . and *everything else* on the other, when compared to the "Big Three."

The specter of "The Big C" seems to hover over nearly everyone these days. There is either a greater incidence of cancer or the diagnostic procedures are more accurate. Probably both. But it always seems to happen to someone else until . . . .

If a growth, spot, mass or other abnormality is noticed, doctors are quick to perform one or more biopsies to determine whether malignancy is present. Because medical science is not infallible, doctors prefer to err on the side of caution and safety. They recommend removal of the offending lump or spot medically, surgically or by radiation.

My first biopsy showed no obvious malignancy. My second biopsy—no malignancy detected. They nevertheless advised surgery. *They did not discover malignancy until surgery!*

I was given that unwelcome news within my first conscious hour in ICU. Now that I've had time to think about it, they should have realized *that was much too soon to tell me.* I was far from emotionally stable and didn't even have the strength for a panic attack. I had to take the news and tuck it away secretly for awhile. Postop pain and weakness were more than enough to deal with at first.

Cancer means that certain cells are out-of-control, in rebellion. For some unknown reason, cells go berserk and grow in a disorderly and chaotic manner. They crowd out healthy cells and rob them of their ability to function normally. Long ago I put myself wholly under God's control, bringing "all that is within me," including my internal organs and a potential malignancy, under His control. Cancer is lack of wholeness. God specializes in making "whole."

Since God led me into surgery, I consider it just as much a healing as instant, miraculous healing would have been. It is God who has given medical science the skill to put me to sleep, cut me open, take the evil out, sew (staple) me up and let God bring me to recovery. *To me, that's a miracle!*

My life is in God's hands, my days on earth are in

God's hands, God's work through me is in His hands. This body is not mine. It is God's. He let my spirit borrow it for a lifetime to do through me what He planned. My body belongs to God by His creation, by His redemption and by my surrender to Him. Therefore, I've already accepted that the maintenance and healing of my body are God's responsibility.

O.K., now I have a personal encounter with "The Big C." I rest my case with God. *One day at a time, Lord, that's all I'm asking from You. I want to do and be what You want, as long as You want.*

Time to take cover

Now that I know I have cancer, I don't feel courageous or heroic—just the opposite. I want to whimper, crawl under the covers and let the world go by.

Since the Lord says "Come unto me," I'm going to take Him up on His invitation. He opens His arms wide and welcomes me to snuggle close to Him like a chick under the wings of a mother hen. Jesus used that illustration to compare His love for Jerusalem and God's chosen people. So did David in the Psalms:

He will cover you with His pinions (feathers), and under His wings you may seek refuge (or trust). (Psalm 91:4)

How precious is Thy lovingkindness, O God! And the children of men take refuge in the shadow of Thy wings." (Psalm 36:7)

Be gracious to me, O God, be gracious to me, for my soul takes refuge in Thee; and in the shadow of Thy wings I will take refuge, until destruction passes by. (Psalm 57:1)

For Thou hast been my help, and in the shadow of Thy wings I sing for joy. My soul clings to Thee. (Psalm 63:7)

That's exactly what I need and want to hear at this moment. The expression "clings to Thee" gives me permission to nestle close. God offers Himself as a place of refuge, safety and protection. He is my hiding place in times of danger, trouble or grief. And in times of crisis, disaster, pain and confusion about what the future may hold for me now. The hymn writer may have had those thoughts from David in mind when he wrote:

Under His wings I am safely abiding,
tho the night deepens and tempests are wild;
Still I can trust Him, I know He will keep me,
He has redeemed me and I am His child. . . .
Under His wings, under His wings,
who from His love can sever?
Under His wings my soul shall abide
safely abide forever.[1]

There's a time to march bravely into battle and a legitimate time to retreat for renewal, to withdraw for restoration. I'm sure the Lord understands my need for "R and R" right now. My Comforter will never leave me; He's called alongside to help, to teach me precious lessons through my physical weakness, to encourage and strengthen, renew and energize me.

After He restores me, I can resume mounting up

with wings as an eagle, running without weariness, walking without fainting. Nevertheless, for now, I don't mind being "chicken" and taking cover under His ample wings.

Miracle-Gro

I'm practicing saying the word "cancer" without swallowing my tongue or gagging. I can finally say it above a whisper and without falsetto.

I also struggle not to go back to kindergarten with my "why-ning" and pestering the Lord to give me reasons. The Lord's eternal protection bubble didn't suddenly burst when cancer invaded my world. They diagnosed one million Americans (not counting the rest of the world) with cancer in one recent year. They tell us that over the years cancer of some kind supposedly will strike three out of four families. There are over 200 forms of cancer.

O.K., so now I, yes *I*, am one of the statistics resulting from planet Earth's fallen condition, polluted atmosphere, pesticides in our food, heredity or any number of unknowns. Nevertheless, I remain absolutely under the protection of the sovereign, tender mercies of God. That's enough for me. I'm not in any condition to cope with the odds on survival rates, possible remissions from chemo, etc.

My bout with cancer may not be a *red light* to stop my life completely (although it may, if God wills). It may be a *yellow caution light* warning me to adjust some things in my life. It's definitely a *green light* signaling me to move on toward spiritual maturity for however long God wants me on Earth.

Green is for "go." Green is also for "growth." Joni Eareckson Tada, a longtime paraplegic, writes in her book *Glorious Intruder,*

> Christians are either growing in the Lord or going backward. That doesn't leave much room in between. It's like true love: it either grows or it begins to die. Love simply can't stand still, and neither can our walk with Christ. . . . To put it another way, the Christian's transmission is equipped with only two gears: Drive and Reverse. There's no such thing as Neutral, let alone Park.[2]

I accept my cancer experience as an accelerated spiritual growth lesson beyond the normal rate of maturing. That extra growth is positive, not negative like cancerous growths. God is speeding up my root growth downward, by taking me through deeper lessons of faith, and upward for lush foliage and abundant fruit.

A TV commercial markets a plant nutrient called "Miracle-Gro." I'm fascinated by the sight of super-size, luscious vegetables and fruits nourished with that amazing plant food. Perhaps God planned my difficult experience to help my spiritual growth with His "miracle-grow."

My goal is not to be a prizewinning tomato, but to win the "prize of the upward call of God in Christ Jesus" (Philippians 3:14).

Hanging on

It's amazing! I can be unconscious in a coma, under anesthesia or almost wiped out with chemo or radiation therapy, but not fainting spiritually!

Physical fainting is losing consciousness. Spiritual fainting is losing the consciousness that God is present, that I am in the hollow of His hand, that He is fully in control. I may reach the point of exhaustion and beyond, of weakness and total depletion of energy, but still be able to *walk in spiritual strength.*

I may slow down from running to walking or even crawling. That may not look like much of a victory. It may not sound spectacular, but it is significant. What must I do to experience this spiritual stamina? "Those who wait for (hope in) the Lord will gain new strength; they will mount up with wings (sprout wings) like eagles, they will run and not get tired, they will walk and not become weary. (Isaiah 40:31 Amplified) Other translators say, "walk and not faint."

I may not be able to fly very high physically.

I may not be able to walk or crawl.

I may not even be able to get out of my bed.

Nevertheless, the Lord promised He would help me, when the only thing I can do is hang on.

But what if I *can't* hang on?

Just before my surgery at the University Hospital in Columbia, Missouri, my relatives took me to Fulton, Missouri where we toured the Westminster Memorial Library. On one level an oversize statue of Winston Churchill took up a whole corner. A small boy about six years old and his mother were looking at the statue when we came in. Since they sculpted Churchill in a seated position, the child took a notion to slip under the ropes and climb up on the immense, stone lap of Churchill.

"Oh, be careful!" cautioned his mother. "Don't fall!"

The youngster replied, "If he was *real*, he'd hold on to me!"

Out of the mouth of babes!

Yes, *real* people care and hold on to children who are in precarious places. *I'm Your child, Lord, and I'm in a precarious place right now. God, You are real! Therefore I know You'll hold on to me when I'm too weak to hold on to You.*

No matter how I prepared myself for this crisis, when I'm in the middle of it, I'm weak and incredibly helpless. I can't hold on to the Lord. I wanted to be strong and brave. I'm not. I feel like a limp, deflated balloon.

I expected to pray a lot while lying in a hospital bed. I memorized Scripture promises. Now I can't recall any of them. I just can't think deep, spiritual thoughts. Or any thoughts at all. What a disappointment!

I'm back to helpless, infant basics without the ability to care for myself. *Lord, please hold on to me. Let me crawl up on Your big lap and snuggle up while You put Your strong arms around me, Abba, Father.*

If hairs, then lungs and heart . . .

"But the very hairs of your head are all numbered. Therefore do not fear; you are of more value than many sparrows" (Matthew 10:30). Jesus did not speak the above words as a parable. I accept them literally. I don't have any reason to spiritualize His statement or take it allegorically. The sparrow comparison is not complimentary to us, even with His quantification of "many." Sparrows were considered the least of all birds.

The statement about hair boggles my mind. I don't know if Jesus meant each hair has a number, or that God keeps track of their total on some Divine Computer—or what. In any case, I suppose His intimate knowledge must include the balding "fallout" and the graying of hair.

Whatever the precise meaning, Jesus declared that *He knows me in intimate detail and He values me.* If my hair matters to Him, as disheveled as it is after surgery, damp and less than fragrant from perspiration and anesthesia, then I don't apologize for putting an appointment with a hairdresser on my most-wanted list after I leave the hospital.

If my hair is important, than so is the condition of my lungs, my heart, my digestive system, my colon, knees and big toe. Whatever abnormalities I or any of the other patients in this hospital have, it obviously matters to God. I can't imagine how that is possible when God has the whole world to manage and the entire universe to keep in order. However, if Jesus said it, I believe it.

How I cling to that marvelous truth!

I lie here watching my heart monitor register my life force. I watch the medication and glucose dripping slowly down the plastic tube into the needle taped to the top of my hand. I sense the shallowness and irregularity of my breathing as my damaged lung struggles to make up for part of its loss, diminished capacity and rerouted connections.

I lie quietly in the presence of God, counting on His life support.

Gazing at my navel

I feel gray and blah, dull and numb, bleak and drab, dismal and somber. *Surely I can't be of use to the Lord in this condition.* I'm glad there isn't a tag clipped somewhere to my case file identifying me as "Christian." That would force me to live up to my spiritual role even under these adverse circumstances.

I feel like drawing into my self-pity shell and licking my wounds, (although I couldn't reach my tongue around to my back with its 12-inch long incision still closed with 40 tiny wire staples). I'm too tired to say anything spiritual or uplifting to anyone. I'm "gazing at my own navel" and wallowing in my gloom.

I feel forgotten and forsaken. Since they gave me the news that I have "The Big C," I'm sure that *if I looked up*, I would see a black cloud over my head like the one in the comic strip that floats above Charlie Brown's little friend wherever he goes.

IF I looked up . . . .

But I haven't been looking up. I've been looking *down*, looking inward. My chin is on my chest. Yes, I know better, but do I always have to act like a child of God? Can't I take a vacation from "being a testimony?" How can I shine for Jesus if my batteries are so low? I'd just as soon leave my light under a bushel or at least under my hospital bed for awhile.

A candy-striper brings me today's mail and the local newspaper. I toss aside the paper. Who cares what's going on in the world? Even war isn't important to me, and certainly not the economy, politics or the latest fashions. I only care about my sorry condition.

A get-well card from a good buddy includes a

Bible verse in her own handwriting: "I sought the Lord, and He answered me, and delivered me from all my fears. *They looked to Him and were radiant,* and their faces shall *never* be ashamed" (Psalm 34:4,5).

Whoa! Awesome! The Holy Spirit must have led her to send me that specific zinger and had her mail the card four days ago to arrive at such a time as this . . . *for my need!*

Can I *never* take the phone off the hook spiritually? Well, the Lord *never* hangs up on me. The Psalmist gave me good advice: "Bless the Lord *at all times;* His praise shall *continually* be in my mouth" (Psalm 34:1). I guess the time I spend in a hospital bed is included in "at all times."

Why am I not radiant? It doesn't take a genius to figure out that I'm not radiating Jesus because *I'm looking at myself* and not *up at Him.* The ball is always in my court. "Unto thee, O Lord, do I *lift up* my soul" (Psalm 25:1). Each time I've sought Him in the past He answered and delivered me. Therefore, I know He can deliver me again.

All right, let's get on with it, Lord. I'm sorry for my senseless withdrawal into my shell. "I trust in Thee; teach me the way in which I should walk; for to Thee I lift up my soul" (Psalm 143:8). *Lord, change my batteries to "Eveready," charged by Your power.*

After all, how much effort does it take to reflect Your light? All I need to do is face in Your direction. If I have Your light within, I glow automatically. I know those sentimental trite expressions: Faith is best seen in dark times; the stars shine brightest on a dark night; when the going gets tough, the tough get going. Nevertheless, Lord, please make such truths real to me. I want to be a good "radiat-er" for You!

A bottle of perfume

The same day a good friend sent me a bottle of obviously costly perfume. Her accompanying note alluded to 2 Corinthians 2:14-16. "Thanks be to God, who always leads us in His triumph in Christ, and manifests through us the sweet aroma of the knowledge of Him in every place. For we are a fragrance of Christ to God among those who are being saved and among those who are perishing; to the one an aroma from death to death, to the other an aroma from life to life. And who is adequate for these things?"

She reminded me that "in every place" does means in the operating room, in my hospital room . . . wherever. This is my second reminder not only to shine for the Lord, but bear His fragrance.

Just a dab of the perfume was enough to offset the antiseptic smell of the room, cover the acrid anesthetic aroma still clinging to me and the odor of perspiration.

Jesus is my fragrance! Although I'm too sick to say much, my attitudes, body language, lack of complaint, patient endurance of pain, appreciation expressed to the hospital staff even for small services, hopefully dispenses a fragrance for Christ.

Lord, please help me be a patient sheep, whose woolly coat gives off Your fragrance, not my wet-sheep odor of grumbles and groans.

I'm God's representative wherever I am—lying down in happy, green pastures of life's pleasant experiences or lying on the white sheets of a hospital bed.

Wonderfully designed

I take my human body for granted until something goes wrong and needs "fixing" by the doctor or an adventure in the hospital.

God did a marvelous job designing the human body. My temporary body house is intricate, extraordinary and magnificent. God thought of absolutely everything. I'm amazed at how well and how long my mortal body keeps running with relatively little body shop repair (except two artificial windows over my eyes from the optometrist). I have my original plumbing, electricity and construction material.

Each day my heart beats approximately 103,689 times, and my blood travels 168,000,000 miles in 24 hours. I breathe 23,040 times a day and never think about it while inhaling 438 cubic feet of air. The average adult supposedly eats 3 1/4 pounds of food and drinks 2.9 pounds of liquids daily. I perspire 1.43 pints on warm days and give off 2.6 degrees Fahrenheit. Is it possible that I speak about 4,800 words a day? Moderately active, I move 750 major muscles. They say that a person moves in his sleep about 25 to 35 times a night.

Incredible and wonderful are not overstatements! God thought up the whole process when He created the first man, and it has been perpetuated ever since. I could never believe that my body "just happened" or evolved by chance from some simple, lower form of life. Psalm 139:13-18 from the Amplified Bible expresses it well:

For You did form my inward parts, You did knit me together in my mother's womb. I will confess and praise You, for You are fearfully wonderful, and for the awful wonder of my birth! Wonderful are Your works, and that my inner self knows right well.

My frame was not hidden from You, when I was being formed in secret and intricately and curiously wrought (as if embroidered with various colors) in the depths of the earth [a region of darkness and mystery].

Your eyes saw my unformed substance, and in Your book all the days of my life were written, before ever they took shape, when as yet there was none of them.

How precious and weighty also are Your thoughts to me, O God! How vast is the sum of them! If I could count them, they are more in number than the sand. When I awoke [could I count to the end] I would still be with You.

Since God wrote all the days of my life in His book before they ever took place, it follows that this surgical episode is a planned chapter, or at least a few paragraphs in my life-book. My ordeal is not God's afterthought but an important part of His plot.

Thank You, Lord for keeping my heart pumping for these long years, and my lungs breathing, and all those unseen, internal parts working automatically! Thank you for the skill You give to surgeons to do the mending when needed.

When God interrupts

God is no pusher. He doesn't invade my life against my will. When I opened my heart and surrendered my life to Him years ago, I gave Him permission to work me over into whatever pattern He originally planned for me.

Year after year, day by day, I've consciously reaffirmed His Lordship to keep running my life:

> *I choose You, Jesus Christ, as Lord of my life. I put myself under Your Master Control. Reign as King of my life with full authority over my body, soul, spirit, mind, emotions and will. Rule over all that I am, all I have, all You have given me. I accept You as Lord over every relationship, responsibility, appetite and ambition.*
>
> *Bring into my life today everything and only whatever and whomever You will—in person, by letter, phone call, thought, impression, prayer, event or circumstance. May I recognize that interruptions and changes are not accidental or incidental, but my opportunities and Your appointments for my good and for Your glory.* [3]

God is not "The Great Puppeteer in the Sky" who pulls strings to either make us jump His way or let us fall in a slump heap. It seems incredible that God chose to give free will to humankind. I can resist God's work in my life but I certainly don't want to!

Sometimes there's a knock on the door of my house that I don't hear. People noises, the blare of TV or the drone of the vacuum cleaner drown it out. Spiritually, I may not hear the Lord knocking at the door of my life wanting to take me through another lesson in His school. Unintentionally, I may hang a "Do Not Disturb" sign on the knob. My life may be so cluttered and busy with good things, even God's things, that I don't hear or pay attention.

At times God may need to drastically interrupt my plans, to switch me to another track. He may use a physical disorder to get my attention.

God is not an intruder in the negative sense. But He is an interrupter, sometimes drawing me back to His perfect plans for me, if I have deviated from them.

Whatever important things I may have on the drawing board of my life pale in comparison to the plan God designed for me. Flat on my back in the hospital, I'm learning to internalize my faith in the sovereignty of God. I willingly acknowledge His continuing Lordship. I want to stay under "Master Command and Control." I don't want to grab the steering wheel from my passenger side.

But Lord, couldn't You have made Your point just as clearly with some handwriting on the wall of my kitchen? Or by speaking through a burning bush in my yard? Did You have to use such a drastic measure as cancer surgery? I think I would have listened to You.

Well, maybe not . . . probably not.

Not in the same way as I hear You now while staring at the ceiling of Room 12 in the surgical wing of University Hospital. ◆

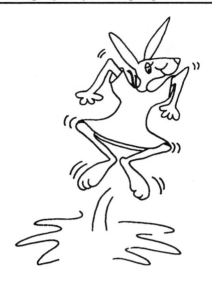

My Personal Workout

1. In what ways can the Lord use my illness to bring glory to Him?

2. What meaningful experiences did I have?

3. How has my pain helped me understand Christ's suffering for me?

4. In what concrete ways have I experienced the comfort of the Lord?

5. What Bible verses are meaningful at this stage of my illness?

6. How have I grown in my relationship with God through my physical problems?

7. How has God seen me through any depression or discouragement?

8. How can I make the prayer "Under the Master's Command and Control"[3] my personal commitment?

9. Consider writing a similar prayer from your own experience.

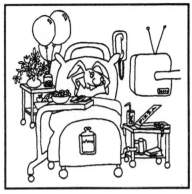

Chapter 9

Dancing in Bed

Acceptance of my situation—for better or worse—is only the first step in moving on through my affliction. Step two? God says it's *joy!*

In various versions, Romans 5:3 is translated "glory in tribulations," "glory in afflictions," "rejoice when we run into problems," "rejoice in our sufferings," "exult in our tribulations," and "boast of our troubles."

The Amplified Bible extends it to the fullest: "Let us also be full of joy now! Let us exult and triumph in our troubles and rejoice in our sufferings."

James 1:2 echoes: "Consider yourselves fortunate when all kinds of trials come your way." Other versions translate it "count it all joy," "consider it complete joy," and "then be happy." The Amplified Bible again gives us tasty dessert to linger over: "Consider it wholly joyful, my brethren, whenever you are enveloped in or encounter trials of any sort, or fall into various temptations."

In Matthew 5:12, Jesus puts His own seal on the response He expects from me when I meet trials of every sort: "Rejoice and be exceeding glad." Other versions are, "be glad and supremely joyful" and "Be happy about it! Be very glad!"

The whole scenario is the exact opposite of my natural inclination when I run headlong into any trial—especially this traumatic illness.

Writing 600 years before Christ, the prophet Habakkuk used similar terms when he faced devastating catastrophes. His whole world, personal and national, was in ruins. But listen to his testimony:

> Though the fig tree should not blossom, and there be no fruit on the vines; though the yield of the olive should fail, and the fields produce no food; though the flock should be cut off from the fold, and there be no cattle in the stalls, *yet I will exult in the Lord, I will rejoice in the God of my salvation.* The Lord God is my strength. (Habakkuk 3:17-19)

The Hebrew term for "exult" means to leap for joy and spin around in the presence of God, to rejoice exceedingly, be highly elated or jubilant. Habakkuk was whooping it up, celebrating, making merry as if it was party time.

Habakkuk was celebrating *because the Lord God was his strength!* His joy in life didn't depend on material things or his own well-being. It was anchored in His God alone. God expects the same response from me under my present circumstances. Can I join Habakkuk on the chorus of that joyful song?

> Yet I will rejoice in the Lord, I will exult in the [victorious] God of my salvation! The Lord is my strength, my personal bravery *and* my invincible army; He makes my feet like hind's feet, and will make me to walk [not to stand still in terror, but to walk] and make [spiritual] progress upon my high places [of trouble, suffering or responsibility]! (^Amplified^)

Since God is my salvation and strength, He wants to teach me how to make *joyful spiritual progress* out of my trial. Even if everything collapses—even if I don't recover—my faith in God shouldn't go down the drain. I can be highly elated, leaping for joy, and spinning around in the presence of God!

I would have to be an acrobat if God expected me to do that literally while lying flat on my back looking at the ceiling. *Nevertheless, I can do it in my spirit!* The nurses won't even know that *I'm dancing in bed,* but God will see me.

And God will be pleased!

Singing in bed

"Sing for joy in the Lord, O you righteous ones; praise is becoming to the upright. . . . Sing praises to Him . . . sing to Him a new song" (Psalm 33:1,3). I do sing, but not in our church choir. Sometimes I sing as I drive alone in my car or when I'm home by myself. However,

I don't think that singing in my hospital room would be appropriate.

My singing will also have to wait because I'm occupied with the basics of learning to breathe with one-third of my lung gone. Under the direction of the respiratory therapist, I use the I.S. (Incentive Spirometer) to clear and expand my lungs. That makes it difficult to sing. Although I can't sing with my voice yet, I desperately need praise songs of deliverance in my distress.

What's this? An "angel" disguised as one of my friends fluttered in with a handful of stereo Christian music cassettes for my headset tape player. God must have sent her! If she brought me a ten course feast of my favorite gourmet foods, I could not appreciate it more! Actually, it *is* a "thanksgiving" feast that I can eat over and over, and it never grows less.

I'm experiencing the verse, "Thou art my hiding place; Thou dost preserve me from trouble; Thou dost surround me with songs of deliverance" (Psalm 32:7). Whatever pain or discomfort I feel, whatever is going on around me, whenever I feel lonely, God's songs are my hiding place. I feel sheltered, preserved and uplifted. "Thou dost *stereo* my ears with songs of deliverance" is my new hospital version of that verse.

Listening to God's Word through Christian music becomes an ideal way to "let the words of Christ dwell in you richly in all wisdom and spiritual understanding." Since the residual anesthesia in my system fuzzes my eyes and mind, reading the Word of God in print is difficult. Music is the ideal way to immerse my spirit in the Word. I discover that my mind can sing along quite harmoniously, and my spirit articulates the words for my soul's benefit. My labored breathing is no hindrance.

When hospital sounds recede at night, God's songs in my ears and in my heart are precious! "The Lord will command His lovingkindness in the daytime, and His song will be with me in the night, a prayer to the God of my life" (Psalm 42:8).

Father knows best

As God's child, sometimes I don't know what I should properly ask my Heavenly Father. My desires run childishly wild. When Jesus' disciples asked for something totally outlandish, Jesus said "You don't know what you are asking." I don't know what's good for me, what would harm me and what is best for God's kingdom. Only my Father knows what I need.

Hundreds of years ago a highly admired Swiss Christian, Niklaus Von der Fluh, expressed his total commitment: "O Lord, take from me what keeps me from Thee; give me what brings me to Thee; and take myself—and give Thyself." God's answer to that prayer is sure to be hazardous to our dream of a pleasure cruise through life.

The words on a bookmark in a get-well card brought me just the right spiritual prescription to understand more clearly some of God's deeper dealings with me:

I asked God for strength to achieve; I was made weak to humbly obey;

I asked for health to do greater things; I was given illness to do better things;

I asked for plenty to be happy; I was given only what I needed to be wise;

I asked for power, fame and praise of men;
I was given weakness to feel the need of
God;
I asked for all things that I might enjoy life,
I was given life that I might enjoy all things;
I got nothing I asked for . . .
but everything I hoped for;
God knows how to answer prayer
better than I know how to ask!
(Author unknown)

The apostle Paul explained that because we don't know how to pray as we ought, God wonderfully provides for our limitation. He promises that the Holy Spirit will take our inappropriate and perhaps mistaken requests and carry them accurately to the Father. The Spirit absolutely and intimately knows the mind of the Father. (Romans 8:26,27)

With a promise so great, I realize that no matter what I pray for, I receive precisely what I need according to the will of God! *Whatever* has come into my life right now is top-of-the-line, the best I could get, "exceedingly abundantly above all we could ask or even think."

Since God's perfect plan for me includes sickness, pain, drastic change of plans, losses, trials and hardships, I accept it from the loving hand of my good God.

After all, my *Father knows best!*

Hear my cry

Lord, thousands of people, patients and staff, must be in this huge hospital. Doubtless many are calling upon You in their desperation and pain. Millions all over the world call upon You at one time. Out of all those voices, how can You hear me, a patient on the fifth floor in Room 12? Nevertheless, I am one of Your children, and I am in distress.

The righteous cry and the Lord hears, and delivers them out of all their troubles. The Lord is near to the brokenhearted, and saves those who are crushed in spirit. Many are the afflictions of the righteous, but the Lord delivers him out of them all. (Psalm 34:17-19)

The ears and eyes of the lifeguard on a beach are trained so acutely that although thousands of bathers combine their voices in a hubbub of noise, he distinguishes a cry of distress.

The Lord is my Shepherd. As His sheep, I am learning to recognize *His voice.* Without question, He knows *my voice.* We are intimate. When a good friend phones me, she usually needs to say only one word, my name. Most of the time I recognize her voice immediately. Therefore, I am confident that when I call upon the Lord in my time of anguish and distress, He hears my cry as if I were His only child. He answers me either with deliverance or by giving me His strength to endure.

I have a remarkable gadget dangling at my bedside. I only need to move my hand slightly to press the button for help. A light instantly flashes at the nurses' control center, and a caring voice asks me over a loudspeaker in my own room, "How may I help you?" I don't even need to wait for someone to come into my room to ask what I need. I can state my need, and they immediately satisfy it.

Lord, You never fail to hear and answer my need.
"I sought the Lord and He answered me. . . . They who
seek the Lord shall not be in want of any good thing"
(Psalm 34:4,10).

Just "what's-her-name"

At the nurses' station they probably refer to me as
"Room 12," or "that post-op lung case," or "Dr. Curtis'
patient." I feel that I'm only a case number, a Social
Security number, a computer account and a hospitalization insurance record. My case folder is getting thicker
by the day, full of information about everything going on
inside and outside of me—things I wouldn't understand
or care to know about. Thank God for people trained to
interpret the data properly.

In some ways, I feel like a nonentity, a zero, but
that's not the way Jesus views me! *I'm not a nobody!* "He
calls His own sheep *by name*" (John 10:3). "The Lord
called me from the womb; from the body of my mother
He *named* me" (Isaiah 49:1).

I'm Not Nobody!

My spirit longs for identity;
The world pressures me
advocating conformity
debasing my personality
championing uniformity.

I abhor the abnormality
of my struggle for individuality

as I stumble around to see
whether I have a special destiny;
I feel swallowed up
in the vanity
of being just a facsimile
of humanity.
But . . .
Jesus knows my name!

I'm not a nonentity!
Before I was born
God predestined me;
Calvary was designed
to set me free
from Satan's captivity
and break me out
of the mold
of anonymity.

I'm not consigned
to the monotony
of homogeneity.
In Jesus, I'm not
a generality;
What a discovery to find out
I'm not generic!
*I'm distinctly ME
and
Jesus knows my name!*[1]

Joni Eareckson Tada affirmed that exciting thought:

> Ah, be encouraged, friend. Even though your name may not roll off the tip of many tongues, God truly remembers who you are. He not only knows your name (first, last, and middle), He knows the exact number of hairs that grace the top of your head. He knows your heart, your worries, your dreams, and your deepest longings. As the Lord told Israel, your name is inscribed on the palms of His hands. Furthermore, there's no "what's-his-name" or "who's-a-which" written down in the Lamb's Book of Life. That's *your* name written there. A name well-known in heaven. And well-loved.[2]

No-name extras

I bless God for the "no-name extras," the ministering angels who attend to me as I lie in my hospital bed. They remind me of the names rapidly scrolled at the end of a television documentary or movie. It's awesome to see the endless number of people who contributed to the production. Each is vital to make the drama successful.

Some do not get credits flashed on the screen. The producer or director hires them to fill in, to provide authentic background or atmosphere. Some appear in mob scenes, street scenes and wars scenes. They fade in and out as needed. Their job is to enhance the scene but not detract from the main performance. In some sense, they are immortalized on the screen. They are "real" people although I don't know their names. Such people seldom say anything. Their job is simply to be what the director wants them to be. He pays them a fair union wage, I suppose, and they have the satisfaction of seeing things go smoothly because they played their assigned part.

Behind the scenes of my hospital drama is a wonderful throng of no-name extras. I met some when I was an outpatient during pre-op: receptionists, paper-work people, "blood takers," x-ray technicians, lab workers, specialists, consultants, radiologists—the number seems legion. It's multiplied on the day of surgery in the operating theater, then in the ICU: nurses, orderlies, more doctors, anesthesiologists and specialists of every kind. I never saw some of them, but their names appear on my bills for services rendered!

For my daily care the no-name dietitians, cooks, medication preparers, cleaning personnel and nursing staff are all available to do things for me that I am helpless to do.

If they wear name tags, I try to call them by name—doctors and nurses, of course. Besides those, I've become acquainted with and love Barbara, the lady who comes daily to empty my waste basket, dust the furniture and clean my bathroom. She told me about her daughter who just went through a divorce. We talked about God together. She is my sister in the Christian faith. Barbara is not a no-name to me.

I'm thankful for the no-name x-ray team who roll in their monster-equipment every morning to take my inward picture. For the orderly who comes to collect my food tray. For the no-name who checks my air-conditioner. For someone who delivers the daily paper to each patient, the television repair man, the helper who comes to put fresh linens on my bed.

I am thankful to God for all of them. *They are not no-names to Him.*

Daily routine

Sarah comes to my hospital room every morning at exactly 8:25. She's a large, middle-aged woman who moves slowly but has a warm smile for me as she sweeps the floor. The first thing she does is tear off yesterday's big-number-date on the wall calendar opposite my bed. Another big number with today's date stares blankly at me. Another day has passed. I have endured another night, thank God.

Soon Carrie arrives with big plastic bags in which to dump my trash. We talk a bit. She is worried about the possibility that war will break out somewhere in the world, since her son is in the army. She lives alone. "Joe sent me money to visit him this winter in California where he's stationed. I love to fly," she confides.

A technician in a white coat saunters in to watch my heart monitor for awhile. He checks the connections on the machine and inspects the tabs on my chest. He pulls down a graphed summary sheet from the past 24 hours of my life and thumbtacks it on my bulletin board for other doctors to look at.

A hospital menu with food choices for the next day lies on my breakfast tray. I have a hard time thinking a day ahead when my selections are restricted to a soft diet. I decide not to decide. Let them bring me whatever they please.

Life-giving, health restoring, medicating IVs continue to slowly drip their contents into my veins.

A plastic I.D. wrist band on which is my name and

the name of my doctor reminds me of who I am. Who am I? I'm a child of God, a daughter of the King, under the care of the Great Physician.

A "Med-Take" computer keyboard and monitor stand on a shelf against the wall opposite my bed. That sophisticated technology replaces the old-fashioned clipboard and charts that hung at the foot of a hospital bed. Each person who checks me, does anything for me, complies with any of my requests, gives me medication or notes my progress or regress in any way stops at the keyboard and records it. All my current life is in its memory system.

"What was all the commotion in the hall last night?" I ask big Dennis, the tall, young male nurse with the cropped red beard who was on duty during the night. He has come to take my morning pulse and temperature.

"Someone died at three a.m. in a room down the hall," he answers, looking sober. "We're here to help, and when we can't, it hurts."

A helicopter whirs closer outside my window. Through the Venetian blind I see it circle and then land near the parking lot. My room on fifth floor overlooks the heli-pad. I wonder what emergency it brings. An accident? A heart attack? A woman in difficult labor? A burn victim? A shooting?

Orderlies change my bed linens. The room is quiet again. Another day begins. God has generously given me another day to live, to breathe, to experience His presence, mercy and love. I'm grateful.

Eventually I'm alone

Visiting hours are over, and my family has gone.

Doctors have made their final rounds. Nurses have "finished" me, checked all my "connections" and brought my pain pill. I've switched off the mini-television at my bedside.

Night settles in. Busy routine hospital sounds become muffled. No noise drifts up from the parking lot five floors below. Slight sounds in the hall are amplified. My heart monitor silently flashes my vital signs. I hear my heart more clearly in my ears as other sounds recede.

I'm alone. *No, not alone,* there are two of us. Always two of us. *God is here* or else my faith is in vain.

"He Himself has said, 'I will never desert you, nor will I ever forsake you'" (Hebrews 13:5). *If You are not here, Jesus, then I am not here. "Christ in you, the hope of glory" is not wishful thinking on my part. Since You live in me, Jesus, I am never alone.*

So let's talk together, Lord, now that we're alone. But . . . I'm tired, so tired. You talk to me, Jesus . . . and I'll just listen. Take my hand, precious Lord. Hold me tightly through the night, until morning light, till dawn . . . either here . . . or "There."

Pleasing to God

How can I please God just lying here in a hospital bed? I'm not used to doing nothing. I'm a "doer," I chafe against passive inactivity. I feel "good for nothing" because I'm not busy serving Him or being productive in some way. I'm not advancing His kingdom. Am I wasting time lying here helpless?

The apostle Paul said, "In everything commending ourselves as servants of God" (2 Corinthians 6:4). Does "in everything" include my languid state of being set aside from active service?

I go over Paul's list of "in everything" in the following six verses to see if I can identify with some of them. "In endurance, in afflictions, in hardship, in distresses, in sleeplessness, in patience, in kindness, in the Holy Spirit, in genuine love, in the power of God, by evil report and good report. . . ." Most of them really do *not* describe active, productive service! Yet they are *experiences* through which I commend myself to the Lord.

Am I behaving as God's good child under my present circumstances? If so, *I am pleasing God.* My productiveness for Him right now is to produce the fruit of the Holy Spirit in my situation. I should bloom wherever He plants me and bear fruit quietly.

I struggle with my inaccurate view of what God wants. I must get over the mistaken idea that my worth to God is dependent on accomplishment—producing something, having something "to show" for the hours of my days and the days of my life.

I am of intrinsic worth to God. His love for me doesn't depend on my constant "doing." He wants me to relax and just "be" what He wants me to be: His obedient child, quietly listening to Him speak through my present experience and enjoying His love. I'm sure that will please Him.

Lifters needed

"They need four lifters in Room 18" blared over the hospital intercom. Apparently they need to move a patient onto a gurney to go . . . somewhere.

The sick fellow who was lowered down through the roof of the house where Jesus was healing people was lucky . . . or blessed! He couldn't get there by himself, but he had four lifters. The Bible doesn't give their names or his. We're not told, but I don't think he hired them. They were probably his good friends. They cared so deeply for him that they devised extreme measures to get him to Jesus.

That's the kind of "lifters" I need. Thank God, I have them— my friends. They come "right through the roof" of the fifth floor. They pick me up and bring me to Jesus by their prayers and their expressed concerns. They cheer me. They help lighten my pain. They are my "support group!" With Paul I can say, "You have done well to share with me in my affliction" (Philippians 4:14).

I'm usually a strong person, self-reliant and independent. I'm the one who gives comfort to others, who bolsters them in their times of trouble. I feel strange to be the one *receiving* comfort. I'm the one who *sends* the get-well cards. I don't think I ever received any.

Suddenly, "It's a-me, O Lord, standin' in the need of prayer," comfort and everything else. That adjustment doesn't come naturally to me. I find it more difficult, even embarrassing, to receive than to give, to let people help me instead of my helping others.

Now I'm vulnerable. I look eagerly for every ounce of comfort available. There's something about a physical illness, especially a major one, that pulls your emotions right to the surface. No "Great Stone Face" heroics are called for in a hospital room.

I pounce on every get-well card the mail person brings, every bouquet of flowers and gift. I treasure every phone call, every visit from my husband, family and friends, every hug, every assurance and word of encouragement. As strong as I've always been, I now lap up each bit of attention, lick my lips and look around for more. I read every note and sentimental, inspirational or humorous verse in every card. Would you believe, I re-read my cards several times?

Since my mind is still sluggish, I can't pray much more than simply call the name "Jesus." So I count heavily on the prayers of my "support group" who touch "the God of all comfort" for me. When a friend phones or writes saying, "I'm praying for you," I hope the person really means it. I cash his spiritual check right away, and count on what it brings from God's storehouse of riches.

One friend put it this way, "When you're flying low physically, hardly skimming the tree tops, that's when the prayers of your friends hold you up and keep you from crashing." I understand that now. The prayers of my friends and concerned others are the wings that bear me up especially when I'm physically weak, in pain, emotionally shaky, and yes, spiritually dry.

I owe a great spiritual debt to those who love me and care about me. They fill my cup which is empty of my own vigor until it "runneth over" with their friendship and prayers. Their encouragement buoys up my depleted strength. My pain is diminished or at least becomes bearable because of their intercession.

God, how can I thank You enough for family and friends and concerned others who are my "lifters!" Now I'm more balanced—I've experienced both sides of the comfort coin: giving comfort and receiving comfort.

Not-so-fringe benefits

When I prepared for surgery, insurance coverage was high on my list of concerns. They asked me for my medical and hospitalization insurance cards at all medical appointments, diagnostic procedures, labs and admissions desks.

Being well-covered was essential. They asked me if I had any supplements to my main insurance. Was I aware of any gaps in my coverage for which I would need additional finances? I checked to see that my premiums were currently paid.

Foremost in my mind was my own welfare. However, I didn't go far in this surgical adventure before I realized that *I'm going through this for the profit of others too.* That's an additional benefit I did not count on—an extended coverage beyond concern for myself. The apostle Paul described it as follows:

> Now I want you to know, brethren, that my circumstances have turned out for the greater progress of the gospel, so that my imprisonment [hospitalization] in the cause of Christ has become well-known to the whole praetorian guard [all the institutional staff] and to everyone else, [my extended influence] and that most of the brethren, trusting in the Lord because of my imprisonment [illness] have far more courage to speak the word of God without fear. (Philippians 1:12-14)

I personalized my situation in brackets in the above verses. I know my prayer partner friends are holding me up from start to finish, but some relatives and friends who seldom talk about praying also tell me they are praying for me. If my illness brings any of them closer to God, it is a worthwhile fringe benefit.

My illness has given me a window of opportunity to share matters of eternity with others without the conversation seeming contrived.

I hope, as Paul did, that what I am going through will in some way result in the furtherance of the gospel. Some who perhaps were "closet Christians," or shy to speak of spiritual matters, now "have far more courage to speak the word of God without fear."

I'm pleased to be forming some brand new friendships and developing some deeper friendships from casual ones.

When technicians and hospital staff make casual, neutral remarks, that gives me a chance to tell them in a natural way that I accept my circumstances as from God. I take the opportunity to tell them that I appreciate their skill and attention. A small seed, nevertheless a seed sown.

As I think about others, my own situation doesn't loom so large. During his excruciating prison experience, Alexander Solzhenitsyn recounted the many painful but valuable things he would have learned in no other way. He wrote, "So, bless you, prison, for having been in my life." When I begin to count my unexpected benefits, I'm beginning to feel likewise.

Campus in the desert

I find myself in the midst of a counselor training program from God. I didn't enroll voluntarily. God paid my tuition and sent me to this campus in the desert. The curriculum is not easy. In my spiritual lab course, He assigned me to find out firsthand what people go through in a major surgery, not only physically, but mentally, emotionally and spiritually.

Formerly, I sympathized with others, but at arms' length. Although I was not intentionally distant, I had never been touched with the feeling of their infirmities or serious physical problems. Empathy has a limit unless we have had at least some similar experiences or have walked with others through them. I sense that God is training me to understand and identify with others, to comfort them in a more meaningful way.

Paul told us plainly in 2 Corinthians 1:3-5, 7(TLB) why God brings us through spiritual desert experiences:

> What a wonderful God we have—he is the Father of our Lord Jesus Christ, the source of every mercy, and the one who so wonderfully comforts and strengthens us in our hardships and trials.
>
> And why does he do this? So that when others are troubled, needing our sympathy and encouragement, we can pass on to them this same help and comfort God has given us.
>
> You can be sure that the more we undergo sufferings for Christ, the more he will shower us with his comfort and encouragement. We are in deep trouble . . . but in our trouble God has comforted us—and this, too, to help you: to show you from our personal experience how God will tenderly comfort you when you undergo these same sufferings. He will give you the strength to endure.

Lord, You have proved so faithful and sufficient for me that I want to recommend You to others. But the hot Saudi sand still burns right through the soles of my hospital slippers and blisters my feet. My spirit is willing—well, sort of—but my flesh is weak.

Please, Lord, guide me through this trackless terrain. Don't let me get lost and disappoint You. Ah, I see Isaiah 58:11 as a signpost! "And the Lord will continually guide you, and satisfy your desire in scorched places, and give strength to your bones; and you will be like a watered garden, and like a spring of water whose waters do not fail."

"Well-watered garden," is translated in some other versions as "ever-flowing spring" and "whose waters never disappoint." *Lord, You've given me plenty of water, running over, to share with others. I don't feel much like an oasis, which, I suppose, is what you mean by "a watered garden." But if You want to bring into my orbit of relationships some other feverish, fatigued travelers on illness roads, here I am. I will invite them to sit with me under Your shadow for shade and rest. I'll share my Jesus-water with those who are thirsty because You've given me more than enough.*

Please help me through this ordeal so I can be a good Water-carrier.

No laughing matter?

Surgery of any kind is no laughing matter. It's serious business. Nevertheless, humorous cards and notes have been like medicine. "A joyful heart makes a cheerful face. . . . A cheerful heart has a continual feast. . . . A joyful heart is good medicine. . . . " (Proverbs 15:13,15; 17:22).

Attitude, the medical profession admits, is a determining factor in recovery. A positive, cheerful outlook apparently affects the restorative bodily processes God built into us. It promotes healing. A joyful heart is like proper nourishment, "a continual feast," though one might still be on a liquid diet! "But you shall serve the Lord your God, and He will bless your bread and your water [soft diet!] and I will remove sickness from your midst" (Exodus 24:25). [Brackets mine]

One of my nurses told me that a cheerful, appreciative patient is much easier to care for. Apparently the reverse of a joyful, cheerful spirit makes recovery more difficult. Medication doesn't work as well in a depressed person or one who complains.

A friend sent me a "funny pill" in the form of a poem, author unknown. After all the pre-op tests and the post-op exams that seem to continue without end, I can identify with the experience.

Pokin' Around

I thought I'd let my doctor check me
'cause I didn't feel quite right.
All those aches and pains annoyed me,
and I couldn't sleep at night.
He could find no real disorder,
but he wouldn't let it rest,
what with Medicare and Blue Cross—
it wouldn't hurt to test.
To the hospital he sent me,
(though I didn't feel that bad).
He arranged for them to give me
every test they ever had!

I was fluoroscoped and cystoscoped,
my aging frame displayed,
stripped upon an ice cold table,
my innards were x-rayed.
I was checked for worms and parasites,
for fungus and the crud,
they pierced me with long needles
sampling my blood.
Doctors checked me over,
probed and pushed and poked around,
and to make sure I was living,
they wired me for sound.
They finally concluded
(their results have filled a page)
that what I have *will* some day kill me—
My affliction is OLD AGE!

Sometimes, of course, the problem *does* turn out to be more than just aging, but God is in control of all that concerns me.

Flip-side definitions

A lighthearted friend sent me a list of "Medical Terms for the Layman" by author unknown. (I'd like to meet "Author Unknown" some day. He or she is a prolific writer!) I could add to this list more new terms I've learned since I started on this surgical adventure. Unfortunately, not all were as funny!

Artery . . . The study of fine paintings
Barium . . . What you do when CPR fails
Caesarean Section . . . A district in Rome

Colic . . . A sheepdog
Coma . . . A punctuation mark
Congenital . . . Friendly
Dilate . . . To live a long time
Fester . . . Quicker
G.I. Series . . . Baseball games between soldiers
Grippe . . . A suitcase
Hangnail . . . A coat hook
Medical staff . . . A doctor's cane
Minor operation . . . Digging for coal
Morbid . . . A higher offer at an auction
Nitrate . . . Lower phone charges than day rate
Node . . . Was aware of
Organic . . . Musical
Outpatient . . . A patient who fainted
Post Operative . . . A letter carrier
Secretion . . . Hiding anything
Serology . . . Study of English Knighthood
Tablet . . . A small table
Tumor . . . An extra pair of something
Urine . . . Opposite of "You're out!"
Varicose Veins . . . Veins that are too close together

Ouch! It hurts to laugh, but it's a sure cure for the blahs. ◆

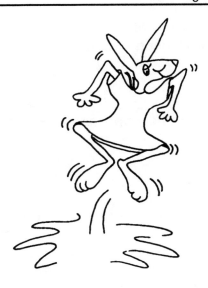

My Personal Workout

1. In what ways might my illness be an answer to my own prayers?

2. What aspects of my hospital journey were the most difficult for me? Why?

3. Are my emotions more sensitive and harder to control during my illness? What emotion seems uppermost in my present situation?

4. How can I express my appreciation for family and friends who have been helpful and solicitous?

5. What specific good has come from my illness experience?

6. Do I have the joy of the Lord on a daily basis no matter how I feel?

7. Can I appreciate humor in spite of my difficult circumstances? Where can I find it?

Part 4

Recovery and Reentry

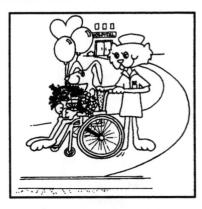

Chapter 10

Is There Life After Hospital?

Finally, the day of my hospital discharge arrives!

Sarah, my faithful room-tidy-up-person tore the last date (for me) off my wall calendar. In anticipation, I didn't select today's lunch from the menu on my tray yesterday! My night nurse made the closing entry on my in-room computer. Before breakfast, my smiling surgeon gave me a list of dos and don'ts. I've thanked every hospital staff person who came by for their "*hospital*-ity."

Staples that held my incision are out, my bandages are checked, and I've been given a fistful of prescriptions. I signed a stack of discharge papers, collected vases and baskets of flowers and put rubber bands around mounds of "get-well" cards. My husband and family have gathered up the hospital "freebies" supplied for my hygiene—toothpaste, talc, lotion. The hospital would trash them anyway.

Still weak and with shaky hands, I managed to open the plastic bag provided at my admittance to hold my real-world clothing. I lay aside my hospital gown at last!

Unlike my hospital gown, my jacket has pockets! I take home invisible pockets full of learning experiences from this hospital classroom.

They are my guarantees that I will never be the same. Not only am I missing some interior body parts, but I've accumulated blessings.

Complying with hospital regulations, they wheelchair me with all my paraphernalia down the elevator to the parking garage. Beyond those doors I will reenter the busy outer atmosphere of my former world.

Thank God, yes, I thank God that hospital doors swing both ways. I've gone in—I'm coming out. Jesus' promise is true: "His sheep go in and out and find pasture." I've done a lot of grazing in the hospital pasture. Now the grass looks greener again on the other side of the hospital fence.

Is there life after hospital? "Today is the first day of the rest of my life." Not just a trite expression, but a truth I eagerly grasp.

None of us knows what amount of the "rest of our life" remains to spend and to invest. Perhaps only an hour or a day. We may have an accident or illness may recur. Will "the rest" be a month, a year, five, ten or more years? Only God, who holds my breath and my beating heart in His hands, knows how long He's planned to give me.

Right now is my only opportunity to be a faithful steward of the rest of my life, however long or short. I am accountable before the Lord *just for today.* Tomorrow is only a series of todays strung across a calendar.

Now that I'm "out of my foxhole" and promoted from a horizontal to a vertical posture, what shall I do to fulfill the concerns about which the Lord spoke so clearly back in Room 12? Can I maintain the intimate, closeness of leaning on Jesus' bosom that sustained me through my hospital adventure? Can I lay aside the dispensable "vain things that charm me most?" Some are legitimate pursuits, but only soap bubbles compared to the "gold, silver and precious stones" that the Lord pointed out to me.

David wrote, "I will come to your temple . . . and fulfill my vows to you—vows my lips promised and my mouth spoke when I was in trouble" (Psalm 66:13,14). Yes, I did make promises to the Lord.

How much can I really change? Many of my life patterns are chiseled in stone. Nevertheless, I know *God can change me* and reshape me by His power and by His Spirit. It doesn't matter how long I've sloshed in ruts or routines which bound me. Thank God, He's still workin' on me!

I'm afraid that I may revert to life as it was and forget what God taught me. I guess that's why God fenced in *another pasture* for me to graze in—a kind of half-way-house as a transition. It is my extended period of *Recovery and Reflection.*

Recovery minefield

I had *hurdles* to jump over when I started on my unfamiliar surgical adventure. They were questions. As I launch into recovery, I find it's like a hazardous *minefield* where I must watch my step.

During the Persian Gulf war, as in most wars, soldiers lost their lives when they stepped on hidden mines in the battlefield. After the cease fire, one of the first demands of our victorious generals was that the enemy must provide maps of the minefields. When you know where the mines are, you won't step on them.

If I know what some perils of my recovery period might be, I can avoid them and "walk circumspectly," as the Bible puts it. Eventually, I can defuse them safely.

● One dangerous hidden mine is my impatience. I'm in such a rush to get well. All those wonderful "get-well *soon*" cards add fuel to my burning impatience. I want to cut short the recuperative stage. But my surgeon cautioned me that it would be a long time before I fully recover, that inside healing will take longer than the outside.

● Discouragement is another mine. In fact, many depression-type mines are scattered throughout my recovery period. All of them are lethal.

● Still another, is the expectation of a smooth, upward path to health. In reality, the recovery road is full of high hills and deep valleys.

● Not being able to understand or accept God's working in my life through this illness is a major mine.

● Other mines? Guilt and disappointment with

myself because of my own poor attitude during recovery.

● A giant mine is my mood swings—not knowing how to handle the tears often close to the surface. This leads to lashing out against others who don't seem to understand my feelings.

● One hazardous mine is too much introspection. Another is insufficient life evaluation and returning to old ruts after God has shown me a higher way.

● The tendency to withdraw and isolate myself from others is a mine ready to explode in my face and maim me.

● Another mine is focusing either too much on my illness or unrealistically denying its seriousness.

● A mine with a double fuse is either expecting or demanding too much attention and help from others, or refusing to accept help from those who sincerely offer it.

● I can easily step on the mine that urges me to take myself too seriously and not relax into the healing balm of humor.

● Self-pity is a deadly mine lying just beneath the surface, ready to detonate at the slightest provocation.

● When I find out that I'm not indispensable, a mine of deflated self-esteem explodes.

● Not recognizing the difference between essential recuperative rest and lazy, degenerating inactivity sets off another mine. It's placed right under my comfortable recliner. Only scheduled times for exercise will help me avoid that hazardous one.

● Black moods of despair, if my illness returns, or if I need to repeat medical or surgical procedures, set off other mines.

● A perilous mine is when I give up without setting

new, realistic life goals or renewing former goals the Lord wants me to continue pursuing.

● The mine of careless physical appearance and attire because I don't feel good about myself is always at hand.

● Many small mines of complaint about my condition are scattered and hidden throughout my recovery desert.

● Most of the above mines are "common to man." I have other personal ones and so do my readers. Some of those suggested above don't explode as readily for me as they might for someone else, but some are like heavy TNT charges.

Let's try to defuse some of our mines together.

Fight back?

"You must fight this thing!" well-meaning friends repeatedly advise me. I thought I settled that hurdle before my surgery. I should only fight against evil—I want to be very sure I'm not fighting against God. That would be a fixed match anyway. I'm a puny, helpless, mortal human. No contest. I don't even want to wrestle with an angel, as Jacob did.

"Disease is evil. Illness is bad. God wouldn't give cancer. Fight it!"

Charles Stanley expanded on the question of whether adversity comes from above or below:

> You may think, *But shouldn't I resist the devil? Shouldn't I stand against him with Scripture and prayer?* Absolutely—when he comes at you *with temptation.* For you know that God has no part in tempting you. But we are not

talking about temptation. The focus is adversity, unexpected tragedy, suffering [when you are sure it is not the direct result of your sin]. . . . It does not make any difference who the *source* is. It matters very little who the *messenger* is. As long as you respond as if it were from God, you will come out a winner.[1]

This illness is *not* good. No question about it. Any physical deviation from normal, healthy or whole can't be good. The promise of God is not that everything happening to me will be good in itself. God's promise means that He is at work *even in* the worst of circumstances to bring good out of them.

The apostle Paul's imprisonment and chains were *not* good in themselves. They were bad, confining and limiting. Nevertheless, he wanted the Christians in Philippi to know that "what has happened to me has really served to advance the gospel" (Philippians 1:13).

My physical ailment is not good either, not standing by itself, but I'm not "standing by myself." I am in Christ, and He is in me. He is Light and wants to shine through me. I am a see-through container like an oil or kerosene lamp. The glass container is nothing by itself. The light inside is important. Through this situation I should let His Light shine through me so others may see that my strength, my coping, my perseverance is from God and not from myself. (2 Corinthians 4:7,11)

The response God wants from me isn't a give-up passivity or a fatalistic sponge thrown in the ring. Nor should I lie down in the road and let an affliction-truck run over me.

God wants my total submission to Him, my endorsement of His sovereign will, my approval of His capable and perfect management of my life.

To go forward with God-given courage, fortified by the grace He abundantly supplies, with tenacious faith and trust in His goodness—that's more pleasing to God than to fight either the symptoms or the core evil. I might pour negative emotions into my bloodstream and body if I have a combative spirit. When I restfully submit to God, I allow my physical body to take its best shot at healing under the Great Physician's supervision.

"Get plenty of rest" is good spiritual therapeutic advice. As I relax, lean back and plug into God's healing power, His presence radiates through me as surely as radiation. If radiation or chemotherapy are called for, or medications prescribed, my restful, accepting spirit and body enhance the treatment's effectiveness.

With the hymn writer I declare:

> Jesus, I am resting, resting,
> in the joy of what Thou art;
> I am finding out the greatness
> of Thy loving heart. . . .
> For by Thy transforming power,
> Thou hast made me whole.[2]

So instead of *fighting,* I'm going to *rest quietly* in God's intensive care for me. I'll let Him drive my life vehicle. If fighting is necessary, I'll let *Him* do it for me. The battle is not mine but the Lord's because it's taking place on His property—me.

A time to weep

I cry occasionally. That surprises me. Tears are not really my style. My illness caught me off guard. I didn't have a chance to work up to the probability of it through gradually failing health. It seemed more like an accident. In the rush of events surrounding surgery and all the in-hospital excitement, my emotions didn't have time to catch up with me. Recovery gives me extended time to think.

I seldom cry from pain or unbearable discomfort. Rather, it is from frustration, panic or confusion. More often, it is for no apparent reason. Sometimes I cry while working through my questions and searching for answers. Sometimes for release when surrendering my struggles and recommitting myself into God's hands.

Crying has two aspects: emotional expression with tears, and crying-prayer. Most "cries" described in the Bible are the latter. God listens to tears, voiced or voiceless, just as He listens to and perfectly understands the "groaning which cannot be uttered" of the Holy Spirit when He intercedes for us. "Crying unto the Lord" is both emotionally therapeutic and spiritually profitable.

What makes us think that a stiff upper lip is the hallmark of a good Christian? Courage isn't stoicism. It's not retreating into a hard shell where it looks as if nothing moves us. Tears are not a sign of weakness.

King Hezekiah, as recorded in 2 Kings 20:1-3, heard the prognosis of his terminal illness. He turned his face to the wall, wept and prayed. I know the feeling. Jeremiah couldn't deliver a message from God without breaking down in tears. King David was every bit a man's man, toughened by military encounters. When David's heart literally overflowed, he wrote again and again:

> In my distress I cried unto the Lord . . .
> My tears have been my food day and night.
> (Psalm 42:3)

> Every night I make my bed swim, I dissolve my couch with my tears . . . The Lord has heard the voice of my weeping. The Lord has heard my supplication. The Lord receives my prayer. (Psalm 6:6,8,9)

Tears themselves are a "voice, a supplication, a prayer." In Psalm 56:8 David tells me that God puts my tears in His bottle and writes them in His book. Whatever that means, I'm grateful for it.

Jesus wept in the face of the death of his close friend, Lazarus, although He Himself was the Resurrection and the Life. He wept over Jerusalem and in the Garden of Gethsemane.

Crying isn't unchristian. Human emotion isn't sissy. On the contrary, bottling up my emotions is as dangerous as an unvented pressure cooker. Shackles on my tears don't help my healing process. Repressed emotions cause stress and worsen my condition with all kinds of physical side effects.

Chuck Swindoll reminds us that one great drawback of our cold, sophisticated society is our reluctance to show tears, that we consider them a sign of weakness and immaturity. He called that silly and unfortunate. The consequence, he said, is that we place "a watchdog named 'restraint'" to guard our hearts. We train this animal to bark, snap and scare away any unexpected guest who seeks entrance.

I often took the leash off this trained-in-restraint watchdog during my illness and recovery. After allowing him to romp freely, granting me the catharsis of tears, he always came back contentedly wagging his tail.

After my tears I am more peaceful, released and fortified to press on.

Among the survivors

Here I am, so far a survivor. I join the crowd that can look back on ordeals, accidents and events that could have been terminal. I am here because God willed it. Acts 17:28 tells me, "in Him we live and move and exist."

Those in this select crowd of survivors can look over their shoulders and recall many narrow escapes: accidents, illnesses, diseases and surgeries. Some of us may have had heart attacks, strokes, contagious diseases and heart bypasses. We may have had pacemakers, transplants and other pseudo parts installed.

Doctors may have kept us alive with life support systems. Part of our crowd may even have been brought back to life when we were literally on our way to our Heavenly Home. Others of us have had cancer and something was removed surgically which could have killed us. Valiant ones are even now undergoing radiation or chemotherapy to keep their condition in check. Others have gone through wars and combat.

In fact, *all of us who are alive are survivors!* We have no idea what "near misses" we've had, which God prevented. Our guardian angels are incredibly alert and capable watch-beings!

Nevertheless, here we are, and here I am. Tim Hansel, a fellow-survivor who lives with constant pain, expresses it for me:

> Do we all have to experience tragedy before we can see life's majesty? I certainly hope not. Perhaps the most important thing I have learned in my journey with pain is the intrinsic value of life itself—the sacredness of each unrepeatable moment. To partake of it is a sheer gift; none of us did anything to deserve it. The most tangible form of grace itself is the substance of our normal everyday life. Perhaps it has been worth all the pain just to learn this one blessed lesson.[3]

Why am I still living today? Just because I'm a tough customer? Am I simply waiting until "my number is up?" As a Christian, I can be sure God's special plan has kept me alive until this moment. Not by accident, nor by my own will or the skills of medical science alone have I lived to see this dawn.

God doesn't keep it a secret why He extends the life of any Christian. I live today to *be* what He wants me to *be*, to *do* what He wants me to *do* and to *speak* what He wants me to *say*. Above all, He has extended my life so I can enjoy *fellowship* with Him. Isaiah 43:21 declares, "The people whom I *formed for Myself*, will declare My praise."

I can't forget for a single moment why I'm still here: God formed me for Himself and created me to praise Him and enjoy fellowship with Him. What an honor! What a privilege!

Jigsaw puzzle

I try to fit my present illness into the puzzle of my life. The longer I live, the more pieces I have to fit in. Children's puzzles are more simple—just ten or so big picture pieces of primary colors with familiar shapes.

My life puzzle now is more like the classic "for ages 12 and up" puzzles with thousands of pieces, complicated scenes of trees and clouds or ocean waves with shades and tones and tiny look-alike pieces. Perhaps it is most like the three-dimensional puzzles which challenge our architectural ability. God hasn't shown me the picture on the cover of the box of my life. If I could see it, I could work my puzzle more easily.

Perhaps the box wasn't sealed and some pieces dropped out, which prevents me from making sense of this situation. Or did this odd piece get mixed in from someone else's life puzzle? God wouldn't let that happen, would He?

As our family worked on puzzles in the past, another person would sometimes come along, look over our shoulder and pick up a piece we were positive didn't fit anywhere. He fit it right in its proper place! Sometimes one of my wise friends will do the same for me in my life-puzzle. Nevertheless, only God knows where He planned my unexpected illness/surgery piece to fit in.

Colossians 2:10 assures me, "and in Him [that is, in Jesus Christ] you have been made complete." Without Christ in control, the puzzle of my life would never make sense. It would always be an unfinished picture, and I would forever be searching frantically for missing pieces. Because I am in Christ, all the pieces *will* eventually fit, and each will be important when the "completed" day arrives. God won't go off and leave me in the middle of a difficult scene. "For I am confident of this very thing, that He who began a good work in you will perfect it until the day of Christ Jesus" (Philippians 1:6).

It's no use for me to try jamming this dark, misfit piece into the place *I think* it might go. The piece, my illness, must be important or God wouldn't have put it in my life-box. I must ask for help over my shoulder from the Lord, the One who designed the original scene. If He doesn't show me right away, I'll put it aside until He does.

The drag of the customary

Now that I'm "back in real life," I share the uneasy feeling that Henri J.M. Nouwen expressed in his book, *Beyond the Mirror.* He had been near death's door after a tragic auto accident.

Again fully immersed in the complexities of daily living, I have to ask myself, "Can I hold on to what I learned?" Recently, someone said to me, "When you were ill you were centered, and the many people who visited you felt a real peace coming from you; but since you are healed and have taken on your many tasks again, much of your old restlessness and anxiety has reappeared."

I have to listen very carefully to these words. Is the glimpse beyond the mirror, real and powerful as it was, not able to keep me focused on God when the demands of our hectic society make themselves felt once again? Can I hold on to the truth of my hospital experience?

At first glance, it seems impossible. How do I keep believing in the unifying, restoring power of God's love when . . . competition, ambition, rivalry and an intense desire for power and prestige seem to fill the air.[4]

As physical strength returns, my hospital adventure begins to take on the distant aura of unreality. I check my scars to be sure it wasn't a dream. I have no diploma or certificate to hold in my hand to prove I passed the test through which God brought me. Most of what I learned from my Teacher was inward, unseen by others.

But *I* know what those things were, and so does the Lord. I don't want to be the same as I was before He enrolled me in His class. My changes aren't outward but inward, spiritual changes. I must work them out in the practical laboratory of my ordinary life.

Daily, ordinary living drags me down to the level of my former life, way back to "B.C."— Before Cancer.

In the midst of my illness I begged the Lord in panic, "O restore me to health and let me live!" (Isaiah 38:16). In my anguish I made some personal promises to Him. From one of the previous wars came the observation, "There are no atheists in foxholes." That is just as true in the operating room or even the waiting room of the doctor's office.

I got through my crisis. God pulled me through. The wind subsided, the storm calmed, and the sun shines again. I slip into "business as usual." Now in recovery, I tend to lose the close connection I forged with the Lord during my fright and anxiety.

Whenever I made a childhood promise to another playmate, I'd seal it with "Cross my heart and hope to die, if I tell a lie!" Then my friend knew I was serious and that I wouldn't break my promise even if someone twisted my arm.

Do I take my promises to others more seriously than those I make to the Lord? I always take Him at His word, surely He takes me at mine. I ask the Holy Spirit to shine His searchlight into the forgotten corners of my illness experience and help me recall clearly all that I promised the Lord in my hospital foxhole in the heat of battle.

My problem is not forgetting my promises to the Lord, but not taking definite, measurable steps toward keeping them. Hopefully, they weren't panic promises, not grandiose fantasies or my own sugarcoated desires. I hope they were realistic and achievable with God's resources. I must keep my promises in line with the uncertainty and brevity of my life, and whether they are truly God's will for me.

I was discharged from my hospital foxhole and mustered out into "civilian life." Lord willing, I will live and take the first steps to keep my promises. So help me God.

God doesn't hold me to *perfection* while I walk about in this mortal body, but He does hold me to perseverance and *progress.*

When trouble isn't bad news

Many things in life are not what they seem. Supposedly, it's all in the eyes of the beholder. When things are going smoothly for me, I don't necessarily grow spiritually. When adversity looms its ugly head, I may be on the growing edge of the most profitable experiences God has planned for me. Robert Schuller expressed it graphically:

> Is the grinding wheel that puts a fresh edge on the knife, or the hoe that breaks up hard soil and plows out weeds, or the sharp knife of the gardener that prunes and snips useless growth to give greater strength to the roots and the trunk, or the north wind that forces the pine to send down roots of steel into granite earth, or the rod in the shepherd's hand that strikes the sheep lest it run blindly off a precipice, or the surgeon's bloody scalpel that cuts away the foreign tumor, or the sculptor's hard hammer and brutal chisel that chip and polish—*are these not all our friends?* [5]

Of course, I must answer *yes,* theoretically. But when each new trouble touches me, I wrestle with it although I know better. I need to be freshly convinced during each new round in the ring. How thankful I am that God is patient with me! Schuller continued to make his point:

When is trouble not trouble, you ask?
When trouble cleans up clutter that you valued
too highly and did not have the courage to
discard or destroy. . . . When trouble teaches
you valuable lessons that you would have been
too blind to see, too arrogant to believe, or too
stubborn to accept any other way than by this
bed of pain; when it slams a door in your face
to force you out of a rut that you would never
have had the courage to leave, and leads you
down a new road through an open door, *then
trouble may be a most valuable experience!*

When trouble creates an opportunity for
you to think, read, write, pray, then trouble is
really a friend who comes to your door wearing
your enemy's jacket! Without trouble we would
be like plants that have sprouted, grown, and
been nurtured in the overprotected shelter of a
hothouse, too tender ever to live in the open![5]

Yes, yes! I'm all ears. Looking back on my own
surgical adventure, I see that God is not really silent to my
questions. I am beginning to hear Him speak through my
circumstances. More from Schuller:

What must you do with your trouble? If
you use your head, there is only one choice
that makes any sense. Turn to God! Years later
you will testify that once you were stopped in
your tracks by what appeared to be an impos-
sibly cruel mountain that blocked your path.
You were mercilessly forced to climb it with
bleeding hands and a breaking heart, until you
reached the summit.

There you found, hidden behind the rugged peak, the greenest little pasture encircling a heaven-pure mountain lake!. . . Let your troubles lead you to Christ, and they will prove to be the best friends you ever had![5]

Laid aside to lay aside

Like it or not, during recovery I learn to lighten my customary load. I need to lay aside, as the Bible terms it, some pursuits and concerns which seemed important. However, with eternity's values in view, they are not. If I don't detach these weights from myself, I may not be able to "obtain the prize of the upward call of God in Christ Jesus" (Philippians 3:14).

A hot air balloon will never mount up if the line is not cut by which it is tethered it to the earth. For the balloon to stay aloft and reach its destination, the crew must either let out more of the hot air supply or throw out more of the ballast (that which they use to weigh it down).

The famous *Double Eagle II* balloon and her crew of three set out for Paris, France from the potato fields of Maine in 1978. Arriving did not come cheaply. To stay aloft on the final leg of their journey, the crew had to throw over the side of the gondola such valuable gear as tape recorders, radios, film, sleeping bags, chairs, most of their water and food and the cooler which contained it. They had to treat even serviceable, necessary things as if they were rubbish to lighten the gondola and reach their destination.

Jesus, speaking of His return in power and glory

in Luke 21:34, warned us to be on guard so our hearts would not get "overloaded" or "weighed down" before His coming. The cares of life were among the dangerous dead weights.

If we are weighed down, we won't be ready for "The Great Liftoff." The Bible says it will "come on us suddenly." Our feet could get stuck in the cement of the cares of this life.

The things which weigh down my heart gondola are usually things seen, temporal things. All of that will eventually be gone. Things eternal and unseen are presently "out of sight," but they are more genuine than things I see. God may be using my illness and surgical adventure to correct my vision closer to His perfect 20-20.

Jesus declared that where my treasure is, my heart will be. Treasures don't have to be costly. Perhaps they are nick-knacks, hobbies, seemingly harmless time-wasters, some relationships, material things and over-indulgences in anything. Work, career or even ministry pursuits sometimes steal our hearts away from Him.

After a devastating earthquake, television cameras focused on a lady grieving over the loss of her lifetime collection of antiques. "Everything that matters to me in life is gone now!" she complained.

Watchman Nee, the well-known Chinese Christian author, wrote, "Is it possible that the precious thing which I am doing 'downstairs in the house,' as it were, might be enough to pin me down—a peg which could hold me to the earth?"

The Lord graciously gives me this time of recovery so that I may examine possible pegs which hold me to the temporal. Either I joyfully and voluntarily lighten my life from those weights, or God may have to take them away. *God gives us all things to richly enjoy, the Bible says, but I must hold them loosely.* I must throw some of them out of my rising balloon like rubbish. With Paul, I'm trying to say, "For [Christ] I have suffered the loss of all things, and count them but rubbish in order that I may gain Christ" (Philippians 3:8).

The ideal time to practice this critical "laying aside" is when I'm laid aside to recover. ◆

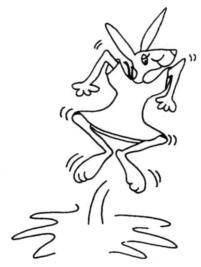

My Personal Workout

1. What were my feelings when I left the hospital?

2. Do I view my recovery period with anticipation or dread? Why?

3. Which of the "mines" listed in the "Recovery minefield" section might I have more difficulty with? (Put an "H" for *Hard* beside those.)

4. Which do I think will be a "piece of cake?" (Put an "E" for *Easy* beside those.) Review your predictions at intervals to see whether they were correct.

5. How do I feel about "fighting" my illness? What other attitude would please God more?

6. Do I have a problem with tears or emotional upsets? Under what circumstances? How can I avoid inflammatory situations?

7. For what specific things am I thankful to God at this point in my recovery?

8. What precise things is God dealing with me about during my illness?

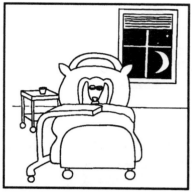

Chapter 11

Downsittings and Uprisings

I am up one day and down the next. One morning I'm happily cruising in the middle of recovery road and by evening I've veered off into a ditch. My surgeon cautioned me that it would take the entire year for full recovery. With my usual bravado, I dismissed such talk as exaggeration. It should be a breeze because I planned to do all the right things. It should be a rapid, smooth, steadily upward road to recovery. A piece of cake!

The first mine exploded! My progress is *not* smoothly uphill. Valleys and hills all the way, full of ruts and bumps which I can't see until I tumble into them. My emotional mood swings demolish my normal shock absorbers. Instead of my usual even keel I feel like a Yo-Yo jerked on a string. I feel guilty because I don't have everything together.

I have to expect emotional mood swings, but I can't predict their arrival during the post surgical or illness recovery period. Even under normal conditions daily life has ebb and flow and ups and downs. My life in Christ is included in that undulation. That does not, however, justify my going on a guilt trip.

The choice is mine. If I'm having a good day, I'll praise God and enjoy my blessing. When I'm in a valley, I must praise the Lord too. A valley isn't a place to *groan* but to *grow.* Through the years I've found that I grow deeper spiritually in the shadows of valleys than when I bask in the sunshine of mountaintops. The Lord can prosper me in both places.

David says, "Thou [Lord] dost know when I sit down and when I rise up; Thou dost understand my thought from afar" (Psalm 139:2). "My downsitting and my uprising" is another translation. The Lord *knows* about my vacillation and *understands* it. I shouldn't be ashamed of normal human experience. God created me with emotions, and He wants to guide me through the rough maze of my long recovery road.

My *downsittings* may have simple physical causes. When I rise rested in the morning, I may be *up* in my spirit and emotions, eager to face the day. Or I may be *down* because I'm unmotivated with nothing special to look forward to. Being physically exhausted and in need of sleep by evening is natural during recovery. That's not depression—that's the human condition.

If I go very long without eating properly or push myself beyond my strength, I use up the reserves of my body and mind. I may need to sit down to a pleasant, nourishing meal with good company. Or perhaps take a nap.

The Lord prescribed a similar treatment for Elijah when he fell into depression after his spectacular success against the priests of Baal. His circuits were overloaded. He had depleted his reserves. He was exhausted. But the Lord didn't lecture Elijah about the evils of depression or slap him on the back with "Cheer up, fellow. Get up and keep running."

As the Great Physician and Divine Nutritionist, God prescribed two cycles of sleep for his recuperation and provided food twice between his siestas. It wasn't junk food either. The angel of the Lord prepared a menu of fresh-baked cake and plenty of water. Not until God satisfied Elijah's physical needs did He send him back into ministry.

Our God is not a slave-driver. He is compassion-ate toward my human frame and deals with my infirmity and weakness in tender mercy and love. I shouldn't be so hard on myself if I can't dash around like a wild horse during my recovery!

My bonus mile

I'm in overtime. I'm enjoying a bonus. The word "bonus" is from the Latin and means "good." It repre-sents something extra, unexpected, a reward, hono-rarium or gift—beyond the norm. The dictionary defines it as something given or paid over and above what is due, more than the agreed arrangement and given free. Generally it's something I don't ask for. Someone in authority gives it to me.

I have a bonus of extended life, however long or

short. Life is so fragile. Any illness or surgery can be life-threatening. Thank God, this time Jesus and I made it through. I don't agree with the term "living on borrowed time." I'm living on *God's predetermined time.*

What am I going to do with my bonus days or years? How shall I redeem, invest, make productive for God and others the extended days of my life?

Has God brought me into recovery without a purpose? Did He heal me only to let me coast along for my own pleasure, just hang around a little longer? Isaiah 38:19 gives me a clue: "It is the living who give thanks to Thee, as I do today." Jesus healed ten men; only one returned to thank Him. Giving thanks is something I should do *daily*, "as I do today."

Here's more good insight from Tim Hansel:

I don't know how much string is left on my ball of twine. There are no guarantees how long any of us will live, but I know full well that I would rather make my days count than merely count my days. I want to live each one of them as close to the core of life as possible, experiencing as much of God and my family and friends as I am capable. Since life is inevitably too short for all of us, I want to enjoy it as much as I can, no matter what the circumstances are.[1]

My desire for my bonus days is to say with the apostle Paul:

> My deep desire and hope is that at all times, and especially just now, I shall be full of courage, so that with my whole being I shall bring honor to Christ, whether I live or die. For what is life? To me, it is Christ.
>
> Death, then, will bring more. But if by continuing to live I can do more worthwhile work, then I am not sure which I should choose. I am pulled in two directions. I want very much to leave this life and be with Christ, which is a far better thing; but for your sake it is much more important that I remain alive.
>
> I am sure of this, and so I know that I will stay. I will stay on with you all, to add to your progress and joy in the faith. . . . (Philippians 1:20-25 GNB)

But Paul, it turned out that your "so I know that I will stay" lasted such a *brief* bonus time, only a few months. Then you left for your eternal reward. Nevertheless, what you accomplished in those *next few months* counted for eternity. You invested your bonus time well and *ran the last mile!* Not knowing God's timing for me, I must do the same.

Bonus blunder

I dread the possibility of following the example of King Hezekiah. What's wrong with imitating such a good man? He was one of the exceptionally fine kings of Judah in the days of Isaiah the prophet. The biblical record in 2 Kings 18-20 and elsewhere lavishly praises His impeccable character and accomplishments for his country.

> He did right in the sight of the Lord . . . he trusted in the Lord . . . after him there was none like him among all the kings of Judah, nor among those who were before him, for he clung to the Lord; he did not depart from following Him, but kept His commandments . . . and the Lord was with him; wherever he went he prospered. . . .

However, in part two of his life the plot thickens. He "became mortally ill" and the prophet Isaiah was sent with a message from the Lord: "Set your house in order, for you shall die and not live." Hezekiah reacted by turning his face to the wall, weeping bitterly, pleading with God to heal him and extend his life. God said O.K. and gave him 15 more years.

Some serious mistakes King Hezekiah made during his bonus period of life nearly canceled out his former good works and brought evil times to his country. He also fathered a son during that period who succeeded him as king. For the next 55 years his son, Manasseh, "did evil in the sight of the Lord," and undid all the good his father had done. He led his people into terrible idolatry and sin and brought God's wrath down on Judah for generations to come.

A quick historical survey and a look at the present reveals examples of people who blew it toward the end of their lives. Sometimes, they begged God for an extension of time after some crisis. In some cases, it might have been better for them to have died, but that's not for any mortal to judge.

Whenever a person goes through an illness, surgery or accident and comes out on the other side, that's
an extension of life. It carries a sober responsibility. The
succeeding days, weeks, months or years should be
precious. We are accountable to invest them for the Lord
as careful stewards. *God forbid that I should "do a
Hezekiah!"*

Health in proper perspective

The question people ask me most frequently
during recovery is, "How are you feeling?" or some
equivalent. That's understandable, especially in the
aftermath of a serious surgical adventure. Those who
inquire aren't asking for a detailed account of ills, pills
and perhaps bills piling up in my mailbox. Usually, they
are only asking a polite question requiring the simple
answer of "Improving" or "Getting along fine." Better yet,
"Thank God, day by day He's helping me make it."

People, even close friends, seldom if ever have
asked me, "Is it well with your soul?" That would be more
meaningful. The health of my soul or spirit should be the
most important concern. What happens to my body is
temporary, at best. Although I am recovering a measure
of physical health, I'm nonetheless "depreciating" day
by day. According to the Second Law of thermodynam-
ics, everything in the material world is degenerating,
winding down, declining, deteriorating. That includes
my mortal body. The Scriptures confirm it but point me
to the happy, spiritual flip side. "Therefore we do not lose
heart, but though our outer man is decaying, yet our
inner man is being renewed day by day" (2 Corinthians
4:16).

My *spiritual health* is top priority. My spirit is the only thing that lasts into eternity. It should be nourished to become robust no matter what happens to my body. The disciple John had it straight when he wrote to his friend Gaius in his third letter, "Dear friend, I am praying that all is well with you and that your *body* is as healthy as I know your *soul* is" (3 John v.2 ᵀᴸᴮ). John already knew that Gaius was in good shape spiritually, so he prayed that Gaius' body might catch up in health to his spirit.

Does my happiness depend on my physical health? So often I've heard the honest comment, "Everything will be fine as long as I have my health." Implying what? That when you lose your health, *you've lost everything?* If we hitch our joy, satisfaction and purpose in life to our good health, it follows that when we've lost some or all of it, we *have* lost everything. That's not true for the Christian.

Moreover, some spiritual illnesses are worse than what may be wrong with my temporary mortal body:

● I may be deaf to God's voice when He wants to get my attention. That's more serious than an *ear* infection or hearing loss.

● I may close my *eyes* to God's truth or His working in my life through this illness. That's worse than cataracts, glaucoma or blindness.

● Not walking with the Lord is worse than bunions, corns or fallen arches on my *feet.*

● Blocked arteries or a *heart attack* are not as serious as the hardening of my heart toward the Lord.

● Worse than *cancer*, is malignant unforgiveness toward someone which consumes my joy in life and metastasizes to other people.

● Not letting God's Holy Spirit guide my *mind* is worse than a brain tumor or Alzheimer's disease.

David prayed with anguish to the Lord in Psalm 51 asking for a complete spiritual overhaul. "Lord, wash me . . . cleanse me . . . purify me . . . create in me a clean heart . . . renew me . . . restore unto me the joy of thy salvation."

That's what my recovery period is all about. The Lord is my Great Physician to whose emergency room I can go when I have either physical or spiritual illnesses. The Lord also practices preventive medicine. He is my day-by-day Health Counselor. He teaches me how to stay spiritually healthy and prevent sicknesses of my heart, life and body.

With the hymn writer I pray, *"Lord Jesus, I long to be perfectly whole."*

Dark moods

If I focus on myself, dark moods of discouragement sometimes descend like murky haze on me. While I'm not a pessimist by temperament, I catch myself imagining "what ifs" about my recovery. That leads me into depression.

According to a legend, the devil once advertised some of his tools for sale at a public auction. Prospective buyers discovered that he labeled one oddly-shaped tool "Not for sale." Asked why, the devil answered, "I can spare some of my other tools, but not that one. It's too useful. It's called *discouragement*. With it I can work my way into hearts that would otherwise be inaccessible. Discouragement opens the door for me to plant anything else I want in a person's heart."

Legitimate physical reasons can lead to discouragement. When the doctor prescribes medications in connection with illness or surgery, the side effects may trigger depression. Some discouragement and depression can, of course, be a direct attack of Satan, and I need to deal with it. His strategy is sneaky.

What is my defense when the evil one comes at me with his favorite tool? Some of what the devil whispers in my ear to discourage me *may be true.* So what? God can deal with the reality of problems and negative circumstances if they arrive. I don't need to go to the corner and welcome them. Jesus said, "Sufficient unto the day is the evil thereof. . . . Therefore take no thought for tomorrow" (Matthew 6:34).

Jesus called the devil a liar and a deceiver. Most of what he tries to plant in my mind is *not true.* In Revelation 12:10 the devil is called "the accuser of our brethren," accusing us before our God day and night. Night time is one of his preferred battle periods. He loves the darkness and tries to manipulate my random thoughts as I lie awake and vulnerable in a dangerous twilight zone.

I can rebuke the enemy by standing on Revelation 12:11, "And they overcame him because of the blood of the Lamb and because of the word of their testimony. . . ." I am no match for the devil in my own strength. I need to put on the whole armor of God so I can stand firm against the "wiles, schemes, strategies, tricks or intrigues" of the devil, as various versions translate Ephesians 6:11.

The Lord gives me a sharp and effective weapon in James 4:7, more useful than the devil's favorite tool.

If I don't use it, I'll lose the battle right from the start. As I get more skilled in the use of this weapon, it can mean the difference between victory and failure when those black, foggy moods start rolling in. The weapon is submission and resistance. They are not opposites.

On my part, I need to do something *toward God* and something *toward the devil.* "*Submit* therefore to God. *Resist* the devil and he will flee from you." That's not complicated, is it? To carry out half the condition is not enough. I must fulfill both requirements. It helps me to pray aloud to the Lord, surrendering myself to Him, submitting my imagination and my circumstances to His control. I sometimes shout aloud at the devil, if I need to, identifying him as real. Nevertheless, he is not nearly as powerful as the Lord within me.

> **Victory is guaranteed because the devil only pretends he is a real lion. He's really a frightened pussy cat. He will dash off with his tail between his legs.**

We may not recognize him because he doesn't have a forked tail, horns or a red suit. He may be wearing one of his disguises as an angel of light—something good or legitimate—but not of God.

The devil tries to convince me to look to the future, but he insists that I put on his special smoky, dark glasses. Through them I visualize increasing physical weakness, possible recurrence of my illness and other "what ifs." Those are not the thoughts *God* wants to plant in my mind. I must deliberately replace the devil's false whisperings with clear promises from God's Word.

"*I have set* the Lord continually before me; because He is at my right hand, I will not be shaken.

Therefore my heart is glad, and my glory rejoices; my
flesh also will dwell securely" (Psalm 16:8,9). Setting the
Lord before me" is an action for which *I* am responsible.
Only then can I expect all those optimistic results to
follow.

Booster tips

We hear so much about "feeling good about
yourself." What does that mean for me as a Christian? It
means the same as for anyone else. I really *do* need
boosters for my self-esteem during recovery.

I saw a television program about cancer patients.
A new nationwide support group has been established to
show women how to use makeup, wigs and choose
fashionable clothing if surgery or cancer treatments
have somewhat altered their normal appearance. That's
great! Doctors claim that we recover more easily when
we maintain healthy self-esteem. Physical appearance
and clothing do play their part.

Whether surgical scars are hidden or visible,
appearance is important both to patients and their
caregivers. Indifference to appearance and careless
hygiene tend to drag one down. I don't have to aim at
qualifying for a beauty contest. I only need to look my
personal best.

Whether lying in bed, wandering around the
house after we're mobile, out for fresh air and exercise
or venturing into public, clean and well-groomed is the
game plan. Around home my outlook becomes more
optimistic when I dress in street clothes rather than
shuffle around in shabby bedroom slippers and tattered
bathrobe.

If I'm not careful, recovery time can cause me to become withdrawn and isolated from "the outside world." It doesn't take long, however, until "cabin fever" may set in, and I *must* get out before I climb the walls to escape. A ride in the car, lunch in town, visiting friends—anything beyond the four walls of the house is helpful.

A great booster is to walk tall in the mall in the company of a cheerful friend or family member. Resting on a mall bench (if I can stand the loud beat of the teen-targeted background music!) and eating a soft cone while watching the passing parade of humanity is definitely therapeutic—or good for a chuckle. While in the mall, an occasional purchase of some new, bright item of apparel goes a long way toward making my day. An appointment for a shampoo and hair styling is a sure-fire elevator for my spirits.

Have all my hospital flowers wilted and my gift house plants died? Then why not buy myself a bunch of flowers or a favorite plant? I can pick out what I like!

Of course, my outward appearance is just veneer. Nevertheless, when the veneer has been somewhat scratched, marred, gouged or "stomped on" through surgery, I should give it special attention. I don't need to feel guilty about taking care of my outward appearance, but happily pursue it, in balance with inward beauty, of course.

How about meeting me at noon tomorrow for lunch at the mall?

Calamities in clusters

Troubles don't seem to arrive one at a time. They hardly ever march in single file. My life may be flowing along quietly without anything alarming happening, then suddenly, like a flash flood, everything breaks loose. Not only for me, but for family and friends, their health, jobs, relationships and circumstances. It seems like a domino effect.

I'm in danger of being swept off my feet. How could so many things happen at once? I don't have the luxury of meeting one thing at a time. Troubles cascade over me like a spring cloudburst with brutal winds and ominous lightning. In the swirling flood, I lash myself securely to God's promises.

The Lord promises that He won't allow anything into my life greater than I can bear, but will provide a way for me to manage it. (1 Corinthians 10:13)

The power of the enemy against my life is limited. God sets the bounds for Satan. He snaps handcuffs on him and keeps the key. Like a police officer in the midst of traffic, God raises His mighty hand with the full authority of the omnipotent Godhead and blows His whistle. That means "Stop! Enough is enough!"

When floods come, the Lord promises to pile sand bags around me to protect me from being overwhelmed by the multitude of devastating happenings. Each promise of God is another heavy sandbag. Evidently, God plays His encouraging background music called "songs of deliverance" while I contend with my clusters of calamities.

Let everyone who is godly pray to Thee in a time when Thou mayest be found; Surely in a flood of great waters they shall not reach him. Thou art my hiding place. Thou dost preserve me from trouble; Thou dost surround me with songs of deliverance. (Psalm 32:6,7)

Save me, O God, for the waters have threatened my life . . . I have come into deep waters, and a flood overflows me . . . May I be delivered from . . . the deep waters. May the flood of water not overflow me, and may the deep not swallow me up. . . .(Psalm 69:1,2,14,15)

God is piling the sandbags higher now. I feel safe. "Thus says the Lord, your creator . . . when you pass through the waters, I will be with you; and through the rivers, they will not overflow you. . . . The Lord . . . makes a way through the sea and a path through the mighty waters. . ." (Isaiah 43:2, 16).

Paul lowered his trusty anchor gleaned from his experience in high water predicaments when waves threatened to overwhelm him. "We are hard pressed on every side, but not crushed; perplexed, but not in despair; persecuted, but not abandoned; struck down, but not destroyed" (2 Corinthians 4:8,9).

The clincher is in verse 18: "So we fix our eyes not on what is seen, but on what is unseen. For what is seen is temporary, but what is unseen is eternal."

What's my part in dealing with this flood of happenings? "Lead me to the rock that is higher than I. . . . He only is my rock and my salvation, my stronghold; I shall not be greatly shaken" (Psalm 61:2; 62:2).

My orders are to cling to Jesus, The Rock, and keep singing God's "Rock music" in the pelting rain and blustery wind *till the storm passes by.*

Downtime

I'm accustomed to mainstream living where all the action is. I thrive on activity, goal-setting and exploring new horizons. I've always been energetic, vigorous and accustomed to motivating others by my strength.

Now I'm on the shore watching other ships pass! They seem to be doing very well without me. I should be happy about that. I've discovered that I'm not as indispensable as I thought, either to others or to God's work.

But I don't like this downtime! A business suffers downtime when equipment breaks and everything grinds to a slowdown or halt. A computer failure immobilizes a bank. Downtime frustrates both customers and employees.

My recovery period seems like useless downtime to me. I get antsy and irritated. The devil assaults me with his deadly weapon of immobility.

Wait a minute. Why do I blame my downtime on the devil? Just because the word is "down" and "up" seems more spiritual? How about, "He makes me *lie down* in green pastures. . . ."? (Psalm 23:2) Why don't I recognize my downtime as the plan of God?

I didn't think I needed quietness to enrich my life just now. To come apart for awhile wasn't even on my prayer list. But I wonder if God might have interrupted my active intentions so that He could accomplish better purposes through me.

I Needed the Quiet

I needed the quiet, so He took me aside
into the shadows where we could confide,
away from the bustle, where all day long
I hurried and worried, active and strong.

I needed quiet, though first I rebelled,
but gently, so gently, the cross He upheld,
and whispered so sweetly of spiritual things.
Weakened in body, my spirit took wings
to heights never dreamed in my active day.
He loved me so greatly He drew me away.

I needed the quiet; no prison my bed,
but a beautiful valley of blessing instead,
a place to grow richer, in Jesus to hide.
I needed the quiet, so He took me aside.
(Author unknown)

A good friend sent me the above poem after my surgery and suggested, knowing my active nature, that I should not only *endure* the quiet and rest but *enjoy* and *profit* from it. "Then they were glad because they were quiet; so He guided them to their desired haven" (Psalm 107:30).

When I drive long distances, I'm inclined to push myself to make time. I usually skip the exits marked "Rest Area." During my recovery, I'm still inclined to step on the accelerator and try to hurry the process. I want quick restoration to health so that I can run again and not become weary, walk and not faint. Mounting up with wings as an eagle really appeals to me. That's my temperament and lifelong habit.

I have forgotten something—the first part of Isaiah 40:31. Perhaps I skip over it because it sounds like a waste of precious time. "They that wait upon the Lord shall renew their strength. . . ." Only after I do the *waiting* should I expect to mount up with wings, run and walk without getting weary.

I tend to think of eagles spending all their time flying with majestic wings outspread, circling high into the clouds. I don't visualize them sitting on favorite high perches and scanning the valley below with their sharp eyes. However, I understand that's exactly what they do much of the time. *They simply wait.* Throughout the darkest night, sometimes even through part of the cold, gray, gloom of morning. Why?

Naturalists tell us that those big birds follow God-given instincts. They rest patiently, renewing their strength from the past day's strenuous activity and flight, storing up vigor and stamina for the coming flight. The eagle waits until the updrafts of warm air currents are just right to bear them up. If the eagle jumped the gun and took off too soon, it would deplete its energy by flapping its great wings for nothing. It couldn't "mount up" without being in the center of thermal currents. Waiting time is not wasted time for the eagle.

Nor for me. God has built into my body, mind and spirit the need for recovering my exhausted resources. If I skipped or cut short the resting period of my recovery, I would flap my wings too soon and flop down into a valley. Through rest I can rebuild what was torn down, recover what was lost, regain what slipped away.

I really do need to refresh what has become stale and revive what is wilting in my spirit and body. I forget that in this surgical adventure I've been through a lot of trauma mentally, emotionally and spiritually as well as physically.

When my *resting* is coupled with *waiting on the Lord,* it revitalizes me spiritually and physically. I'm learning to relax in Jesus. With David I pray, "Restore to me the joy of Thy salvation" (Psalm 51:12).

I finally learned from driving experience that "Rest Area Ahead" is not a casual, optional suggestion. It's an indispensable invitation. So is waiting on the Lord during the *Rest Areas* along my road to recovery. If this provision is "for the birds," the big eagles, no wonder I need it too. Didn't Jesus say, "You are of much more value than many sparrows"? ◆

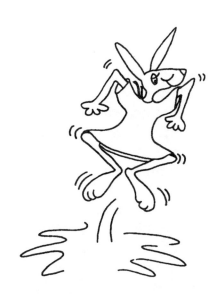

My Personal Workout

1. What kind of emotional ups and downs have I experienced during recovery? When do my "downs" occur, and what can I do about them? How have I appropriated God's help in such periods?

2. How could I conceivably "blow it" during whatever extended period of life God gives me? What must I be especially watchful about?

3. Do I value my health above all things? How would an eternal viewpoint affect my perspective?

4. Has the devil whispered any false things to me? Does James 4:7 really work for me?

5. On a scale of 1-10, (10 = perfect) how do I rate my:
   a. Grooming and appearance
   b. Socializing away from home, if I'm able
   c. Exercise, as prescribed
   d. Proper nutrition and diet restrictions
   e. Taking my medications
   f. Positive attitude
   g. Patience and kindness toward caregivers

6. Have I used my enforced solitude and "downtime" in a spiritually productive way?

7. Do I take time to listen to God quietly? What is He saying to me?

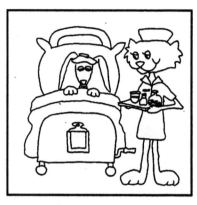

Chapter 12

Oil In My Water

Before my surgical experience, I complained because it looked as if my green pastures were becoming a desert, and the still waters of my life were contaminated. I indulged in pitiful "if only" speculations.

If only I wasn't ill, I could accomplish more of my goals. *If only* I didn't have to take time out for surgery, I could serve the Lord better. Now I complain *if only* my recovery wasn't so slow, *if only* it wasn't such a waste of time. It really sets me back.

Since the Persian Gulf War, most people know where Kuwait is. A generation or so ago, few knew or cared. That postage stamp size country was desolate and inhabited mostly by poor, nearly destitute, Bedouin tent-dwelling tribesmen who were sheep and goat herders. They lived under pathetic conditions. As if their situation wasn't bad enough, contaminated water threatened their livelihood.

They complained, "*If only* oil wasn't in the water of our wells and rivers, our animals could safely drink and perhaps we could survive."

Suddenly they discovered they were incredibly rich because of the plentiful oil beneath the surface of their sand! Kuwait became one of the wealthiest countries in the world. Lavish palaces replaced grubby tents.

From the vantage point of my surgery and recovery in process, I'm beginning to see that God gave me rich oil resources under the surface of what I thought was my barren desert.

Despite the trauma, difficulties, changes of my plans and "time off" from my personal enterprises, the experience is becoming *a palm-treed oasis!* I knew God wouldn't allow anything into my life that wasn't for my good and for His glory. He is proving that! How can something intrinsically bad turn into benefit? God specializes in doing that. Romans 8:28 spells it out: "We are assured *and* know that all things work together *and* are [fitting into a plan] for good for those who love God and are called according to [His] design *and* purpose". (Amplified)

No exceptions. Not a glib platitude. A bed rock truth of God. If any situation, even an adverse, painful one, presses you closer to Him, *it is good*. It may not be an event I have control over, but I can control my response.

If I accept it from the hand of my loving Lord, grimy crude oil can turn to gold!

Mental control panel

My mind plays a major part in my sickness/ wellness adventure. Sometimes it's my friend, sometimes my enemy, depending on which button I push on my mental control panel.

The human mind is one of our most complex and miraculous parts. No computer can match it no matter how sophisticated its circuitry. They tell us that even the most brilliant people use only a small portion of their brain potential. Our minds have hidden and perhaps untapped functions.

I've heard that the average person has *10,000 thoughts a day.* How can they monitor that? Apparently my mind is never blank, but continues to function even during sleep. From the day of my birth, my mind runs a marathon race to gain knowledge, understand, create, dream and accomplish marvelous things during my lifetime. Or to crash land its precious cargo like a plane out-of-control.

Other people and forces try to control our minds. These days "Mind Control" teachers who peddle New Age Eastern philosophy under the guise of success or motivation seminars deceive people and lead them into dangerous occult practices. The battle for our minds is fierce, including attacks from unseen spiritual forces.

God doesn't leave His children without anchors in this churning sea of confusion. The Bible has much to teach me about mind control. How desperately I need it during my time of illness and recovery! My thoughts strongly affect my healing process. Paul instructs: "Casting down imaginations and every high thing that exalts itself against the knowledge of God . . . bring every thought captive to the obedience of Christ" (2 Corinthians 10:5).

The uncontrolled thoughts and imaginations of my mind are like illusive butterflies. They are inclined to randomly flutter around, drifting with any whiff of wind. They directly relate to the butterflies in my stomach. Their breeding place is in my emotions, and my thinking spills its contents into my emotions. God's Word so often links the two: "your hearts and minds."

> And the peace of God, which surpasses all comprehension, shall guard *your hearts and your minds* in Christ Jesus. . . . Whatever is true, whatever is honorable, whatever is right, whatever is pure, whatever is lovely, whatever is of good repute, if there is any excellence and if anything worthy of praise, let your mind dwell on these things. (Philippians 4:7,8)

Obviously, *I can choose* what I allow my mind to think about because *my will* is at the steering wheel. Someone is going to control my mind whether it's me, others, Satan or Christ. My mind doesn't float around in neutral. I'm seat-belted in the driver's seat. I *can* control the direction of my thoughts. Before my surgery, I began to practice with the butterfly net. Now, during recovery, more than ever I need to capture my thoughts and bring them into submission to Christ.

The Scripture tells me to "let the mind of Christ" be in me. That will fill all the space and crowd out unworthy thoughts and anxieties. The Lord is the *Divine Mind-Reader*. Psalms 94, 139, Isaiah 66 and Hebrews 4 assure me the Lord knows the thoughts of man, even the intentions of the heart and understands them afar off. I can hide nothing. During the lifetime of Jesus, the Bible recorded that Jesus knew what people were thinking. Therefore, the Lord knows how wild my thoughts and imaginations concerning my illness become if I don't shackle them to Him.

The button I must push on my mental control panel is marked *JESUS.* That will summon the Lord's security guard named "Peace." God assigns him to pace back and forth to "garrison and mount guard over your hearts and minds in Christ Jesus" (Philippians 4:7 Amplified).

"Peace" is perfectly capable of guarding 10,000 thought-prisoners!

Binocular vision

If I look through the larger lenses on my binoculars and focus on an object or scene, things seem smaller. If I turn them around and look through the smaller lenses, everything seems larger. The object hasn't changed size; it is only an illusion.

If I focus on my problem and my illness, magnifying it above everything else in my life, highlighting its significance, it looms larger than I can handle. It is exaggerated all out of proportion to its importance.

If I concentrate on the Lord, lifting Him up, accenting His greatness, emphasizing His control of my life and my circumstances, I'm looking through the lenses of my spiritual binoculars that magnify. If I'm looking at God, that's the proper end to look through. I can't amplify God to make Him any greater than He is. Almighty God is so great already that He fills the universe! "Great is the Lord, and greatly to be praised!" I'm simply recognizing and affirming His greatness and His ability to handle me and my situation.

By fixing my attention on myself, I exaggerate my own importance. Yes, I'm special to God. I agree with Job when he marveled why God would pay attention to mere human beings. "What is man that thou dost magnify him, and that thou art concerned about him?" (Job 7:17) It's amazing that God cares about me when He has so many weighty, international and universal things on His mind. However, I shouldn't get puffed up to think of myself more highly than I ought to think. (Romans 12:3) My attention should be on God, not on myself.

"O magnify the Lord with me, and let us exalt His name together" (Psalm 34:3). Of course I can magnify the Lord by myself. Nevertheless, if I acknowledge His greatness before others or in the company of others, praising Him with other believers, I glorify God in a larger way. There's something about corporate worship that builds me up and makes my faith stronger than going it alone.

"Let all who seek Thee rejoice and be glad in Thee; Let those who love Thy salvation say continually, 'The Lord be magnified!'" (Psalm 40:16). I decide which end of the binoculars to look through. I can choose what to diminish or magnify.

Search me, O Lord

When things were happening thick and fast in the emergency surrounding my surgery, I didn't take time to deal seriously with the long range implications of my life. I had enough to do to survive the present. I floated along trying to cope with one thing at a time as it came at me.

Now I find myself in the long haul of recovery with time to consider weighty life issues. I'm beginning to reflect, to soberly self-examine my life. I must attempt that evaluation with the Lord who can give me insight and courage to search out what He wants me to see. He brings to my mind some very heavy questions that will take time to answer.

It's urgent to measure the days ahead, although I can't know how many there are. Only God knows. Whatever their number, I feel a greater compulsion to redeem the days I have left. However long or short my life span will be, my days are less than when I started.

In the quietness and open-end time of my recovery, I drafted some questions to help me think and pray through my journey for the coming days. Because this is an extended "Personal Workout," I listed those questions in *"The Back of the Book"* section under the heading, *Take Time Out.* [1]

There are no right or wrong answers. Your answers are private, as mine are. They are not meant to discourage you if you see poor progress or make you too proud as you consider your successes. I didn't whiz through them in an hour or at one sitting. I confess that I don't know how to answer some. The questions reach deep into my soul. Because there are 31, you may like to do as I did and consider one question a day for a month in your quiet time. You may write your answers so you can review them from time to time at other stages of your life.

"Search me, O God, and know my heart; Try me and know my anxious thoughts; and see if there be any hurtful way in me, and lead me in the everlasting way" (Psalm 139:23,24).

Fresh, daily delivery

I thought I could pole vault my recovery time in one great leap. Instead, I'm crawling. I wanted to fly right away—but I can barely walk. How long before I will feel normal again? My typical impatience rears its ugly head.

I've rediscovered a marvelously unlimited promise from God. "As your days, so shall your strength be" (Deuteronomy 33:25 ᴿˢⱽ).

Other translations are, "may your strength be equal to your days" (ᴹᴸ) and "may your strength match the length of your days" (ᵀᴸᴮ). An intriguing translation is "according to your days, so shall your leisurely walk be." I'm accustomed to running. I'm impatient with a treadmill or stationery exercise bike because it doesn't go anywhere. This promise is like new marching orders: I'm to take it easy, stroll through this day with my hand in God's strong hand, and whatever it holds, God and I will be equal to it.

Each day, born afresh, brings God's supply of new strength so I can tackle whatever problems come my way. The Lord wants me to be nearsighted regarding trust—one day at a time is enough for me to take on. I'll leave the long haul to my omniscient Lord who has all the details worked out in advance.

Jesus commanded, not suggested, that I should not to be anxious about tomorrow. I can't live tomorrow ahead of time. Worrying about the unknown only stirs up my fears. I really can't call on tomorrow's provision of strength because it isn't available to me yet. I must open a new box of God's marvelous grace each morning. It is always fresh, always sufficient.

Yesterday's supply of grace is already spent.

Today I must use what is available for me today. I receive
God's strength and wisdom in direct proportion to *this
day's need.* I can't store up or refrigerate God's grace. It's
delivered "new every morning." Like manna provided by
God in the wilderness for the people of Israel, it falls
afresh into my life daily.

Never overdrawn

I have difficulty balancing my checkbook even for
the few checks I write each month. My balance seldom
agrees with the bank's, and they frequently have to
correct my math. The bank statement always seems
accurate. Occasionally I overdraw and the bank charges
an astronomical and painful service charge. It surprises
and delights me when my monthly statement informs me
that I have more money in my account than I thought!

Whenever my day requires it, however, I always
have more of God's grace and strength. He doesn't give
me barely enough; my generous Lord gives me *more
than enough!*

The hymn based on James 4:6 encourages me:

He giveth more grace when the burden
grows greater;
He sendeth more strength when the labors
increase.
To added affliction, He addeth His mercy;
To multiplied trials, His multiplied peace.
His love has no limit; His grace has no
measure;
His power has no boundary known unto
men.

For out of His infinite riches in Jesus,
He giveth, and giveth, and giveth again.[2]

    The Lord invites me to look in my spiritual check-book and be surprised at the bountiful balance. Why do I have such an abundance? My account is in God's name, and He signed a blank check for me. God deposited more than I could ever use. After all, I have His promise from Philippians 4:9, "My God shall supply all your needs according to His riches in glory in Christ Jesus."
    No economic crash can wipe God's riches out. His bank won't go under and He won't need a government bailout. His precious commodities will never devaluate. His oil well can't go dry.

      When we have exhausted our store of
endurance;
      When our strength has failed 'ere the day
is half done;
      When we reach the end of our hoarded
resources,
      our Father's full giving is only begun.[2]

    At times during my recovery I *have* reached my limit before noon. I've come to the end of my rope. Nevertheless, "out of His infinite riches in Jesus, He giveth, and giveth and giveth again." I can never overdraw my spiritual checkbook! Jesus and I are going to make it after all!

Counting what's absent

    Shall I thank God for *nothing?* I should and I will.

This day I thank God for any "a o" He is giving me. "A o"? I refer to the "*absence of* something."

If I don't hurt right now, I thank God for the absence of pain. If I have a good report on a test or x-ray, I thank God for the absence of an immediate problem. If I can put my feet on the floor in the morning and get dressed, I thank God for absence of paralysis. If I am strong enough to continue my work and responsibilities, I thank God for absence of weakness. If I can enjoy my nutritious food, I thank God for absence of nausea or indigestion. If I can pay for my medical bills and medication, I thank God for absence of debt. If I am joyful in the Lord, I thank God for absence of discouragement or depression.

Day by day I total up every "a o" and praise God, counting the things that are *not* happening to me, naming them one by one. "*In everything* by prayer and supplication with thanksgiving. . . ." (Philippians 4:6) The "everything" for which I should give thanks is all-inclusive.

God is my Chief Dietitian. Would I dare refuse anything that appears on my life tray from Him? Since I'm under God's direct management, He only serves me the best menu and the most nourishing spiritual food. *Lord, give me the appetite and obedience to eat it, if by chance it tastes bitter!*

I don't take for granted any crumb of favorable news about my condition. Favorable news includes a test which shows nothing wrong or a clear x-ray. I feel like doing what the one healed leper did in gratitude—he praised God in a loud voice, threw himself at Jesus' feet and thanked him. I keep reminding myself of God's gracious tokens in the things which *don't* happen to me.

Cleared for takeoff

Over the loudspeaker the jetliner pilot finally announces "Cleared for takeoff!" Engines rev up to full power, and the plane roars down the runway gathering speed. Soon we're airborne. The flight crew and ground crew take as much time as they need to meticulously check all systems so we can safely take off. Many lives depend on their careful attention to details.

I've been on scores of flights, many across oceans and around the world. The exact departure time is always uncertain, hinging on the final word from the control tower. Nevertheless, all systems must remain ready for momentary takeoff.

My physical crisis caught me by surprise. I was in the midst of worthwhile, ambitious, busy projects. I spent almost no time thinking about getting my life "cleared for takeoff." Not yet.

The rich farmer introduced in Jesus' parable in Luke 12 was planning to expand and modernize his already thriving business enterprises. He thought he had it made for a promising, carefree future. He had ambitious building plans after which he expected to retire and "take his ease." He probably looked forward to indulging in the gourmet foods of that day and didn't plan to give a thought to cholesterol. He would drink to his heart's content with his good buddies and live high on easy street "for many years to come." He didn't think about his mortality or God. The record doesn't tell us how old he was.

Evidently, he did not prepare a Last Will and Testament because God said to him, "Now who will own what you have prepared?" That very night, "in the midst of" his enthusiastic, long term dreams he died. Jesus minced no words. He called the man a fool.

Because I am "in the midst of" what I think are important endeavors, like that gentleman farmer, there is no guarantee God won't break in with a medical crisis, accident or even a final Home Call. James cautioned:

> Come now, you who say, "Today or tomorrow, we shall go to such and such a city, and spend a year there and engage in business and make a profit." Yet you do not know what your life will be like tomorrow. You are just a vapor that appears for a little while and then vanishes away. Instead, you ought to say, "If the Lord wills, we shall live and also do this or that." (James 4:13-15)

God may be graciously giving me some extended time to "set my house in order." Each additional day is a priceless gift which I gratefully receive from the hand of my God.

I need to give some serious thought to "set my house in order." As to the state of my immortal spirit, it is well with my soul. I'm trusting in Jesus Christ for my eternal future. To maintain a close relationship with Him must be my daily priority.

Beyond that, I have a lot of unfinished earthly business. I need to pull in loose ends everywhere. I should update my Last Will, decide on the disposition of the few, but important to me, possessions. I should spend more quality time with family and friends. I should speak in love the things I should speak. I should express appreciation to others, encouraging them, affirming, loving them *and telling them so.* I should let them understand that the source of my life's joy and purpose is in Jesus, as I long for theirs to be. I should get in touch with friends whom I've known through the years to express again my care and regard for them.

Then I need to deal with some common, everyday things like long-neglected closets, drawers, shelves and storage areas. When I regain strength, I want to get my hands on those accumulated whatevers to weed them out, give them away or throw them out.

"Cleared" is the key. Rule of thumb: if I haven't used it in the past five years, chances are I won't in the next 50! If I "take off" for heaven tomorrow, what would anyone do with all my *stuff?* I shouldn't burden others.

My goal is "loose living" in the sense of owning only what I really need and not accumulating excess baggage—back to basics. Yes, "God has given us richly all things to enjoy," the Scripture says. I want to enjoy everything, appreciate material things but not necessarily own them or grip them tightly.

Hurrah! I feel more free already! I could live another hundred years like this!

"W y d s" that count

Most of my recovery time is made up of ordinary "w y d s"—"whatever you do". It amazes me that God is actually concerned about all the common things of my life. He wants me to do them all for Him.

A "w y d" is whatever fills the hours of my day and night. It is absolutely *anything* I do—the commonplace, mundane routines of life. If I doubt that all those seemingly insignificant things mean anything to God, His Word declares they do:

Whether, then, you eat or drink or *whatever you do*, do all to the glory of God. And *whatever you do* in word or in deed, do all in the name of the Lord Jesus, giving thanks through Him to God the Father . . . so that in all things God may be glorified through Jesus Christ, to whom belongs the glory and dominion forever and ever. Amen. (1 Corinthians 10:31; Colossians 3:17; 1 Peter 4:11)

If I take these truths literally, it means that not only when I read the Bible, pray, worship or do so-called Christian service do I glorify the Lord. *Anything* at all that I do during 24 hours of daily living can glorify God.

A "w y d" is another way of saying "all your ways." As the Bible instructs, "*In all your ways* acknowledge Him [the Lord] and He shall direct your paths" (Proverbs 3:6).

If I'm still thinking of the *big* things, the context of the verses above is eating and drinking. By implication, it would include the ordinary, neutral things like getting up, brushing teeth, attending to my appearance, exercising, listening, talking, resting, reading, phoning and thinking.

At this point in my recovery, "w y d" means taking my medications, cooking and eating nourishing foods, not overstepping dietary restrictions, forcing myself, if necessary, to take prescribed exercises, resting whether I feel like it or not, going for my periodic x-rays or medical checkups and chemo or other therapy appointments. It would also include submitting my private thoughts and anxieties to God, watching my attitude toward everyday tedium, irritations, pain or discomfort and maintaining a thankful heart *whatever my progress.*

How can such common things glorify God? I don't understand it any more than I understand why God is so intimately involved in my life that He even numbers the hairs of my head. It blows me away to think about that, but it does give me a new perspective on my repetitious and often tedious daily classroom assignments of recovery.

God says He cares *what my motive is when I do them.* He wants me to do everything *for Him.* He accepts such ordinary acts as my praise to Him. That's awesome!

Well, in Your name, Jesus, and for Your glory, I'm going for my fresh air walk. You've said my body is the temple of Your Holy Spirit, therefore, I must keep it in good condition. It won't be a monotonous assignment— it will be a praise performance!

I'm getting stomped

Some days, for no apparent reason, I'm depressed and discouraged. A friend gave me a large, glossy poster in full color—the head of a long-eared, mournful hound dog with soulful eyes. The caption reads, "I know I'm victorious, Lord, but it sure feels like I'm getting stomped!" *That's me, O Lord.*

A pit is a deep hole into which one has to be let down or thrown in. I have a lot of letdowns that throw me into the pits: the letdown of a crisis passed, whether the news was good or bad; the letdown of my limited strength after a lifetime of robust health; the letdown of slow recovery. I want to fly, but I've slowed to barely a walk.

I feel lethargic from head to toe like a stagnant pond. I understand that anesthesia sometimes takes months to work its way out of the body after surgery. Medications often cause depression. The doctor told me to remember that I have a battered system, inside and out, as a result of surgery. My mind is sluggish, as if it went on vacation but without the revitalizing benefits of a holiday. "I am counted with them that go down into the pit: I am as a man that hath no strength" (Psalm 88:4 ᴷᴶᵛ).

I also have valid reasons for *not* being in the pits. Surgery *is* behind me and I *am* alive and recovering. "O Lord, thou hast brought up my soul from the grave: thou hast kept me alive, *that I should not go down to the pit"* (Psalm 30:3 ᴷᴶᵛ).

It must be my spiritual life that needs recharging. I'd like new power and joy and praise to flow through all the pipes of my life. *Lord, tune me to Your perfect pitch.*

The direction out of any pit is up. The rungs of the ladder upward are faith and trust in God—as they always are. I must begin by looking upward out of the darkness of my pit into the shining face of Jesus. "O God, restore us, and cause Thy face to shine upon us, and we will be saved." Psalm 80 repeats that refrain three times.

Lord, bring me out of this emotional depression pit and anchor me on higher ground. The sides are slippery. I'm almost out and then I slip back in. I must claim Your promises:

> Because he has loved Me, therefore I will deliver him; I will set him securely on high, because he has known My name. (Psalm 90:14)

> He brought me up also out of an horrible pit, out of the miry clay, and set my feet upon a rock, and established my goings. (Psalm 40:2 ᴷᴶᵛ)

Lord, thank You for pushing me up from behind, while dropping a heavenly rope down and pulling me out!

Free medication

The price of medications these days has skyrocketed! This is especially staggering if the word from my white-coated medicine man is, "You'll have to take these medications daily for the rest of your life." Worse yet if your medical insurance doesn't cover such ingested goodies.

One medicine, thankfully, is not only inexpensive but free! It is *laughter,* and the prescription is from the Bible. "A cheerful heart is good medicine" (Proverbs 17:22).

Although they do not know exactly how it works, doctors tell us that such things as exercise and laughter release positive health into our bloodstream. Humor can break life into little pieces and make it liveable. Laughter adds richness, texture and color to otherwise ordinary days. It is a gift, a choice, a discipline and an art.

Life is really rather funny despite many tragic realities, if we only give it a chance. I enjoy laughing. I believe laughter is a sacred sound to our God. Countless moments of serendipity are constantly beckoning us, inviting us to participate, if we have eyes to see, ears to hear, and hearts to respond.

Everyday life has its own hidden comedy. When we can laugh at ourselves, our situations and the life around us, it literally produces physiological and chemical changes in our bodies that bring about a sense of vitality, health, and even healing. [3]

Was the above dished out by a healthy, pain-free, happy-go-lucky advisor? Hardly. Tim Hansel, whom I have quoted before, wrote it. For more than 20 years Tim has lived with continual physical pain, the result of a climbing mishap in the Sierras.

Since the physical and emotional results of hearty laughter are so beneficial, I should go looking for laughter or create it myself instead of waiting for it to find me. If I take myself too seriously, no matter what the prognosis of my condition, it can be counterproductive.

Whether it's curling up in a recliner to read one of the many humorous Erma Bombeck books, watching a sit-com on television, renting a comedy from the video store, visiting with a good buddy who has a sense of humor or chatting on the phone with a known-to-be-merry friend, I'm going for it. I'm going to "double my pleasure and double my fun" by sharing my laughter with someone else who could use some lightening up. I'm always eager to take advantage of "freebies."

Meat tenderizer

The term doesn't sound very spiritual, but I'm beginning to realize that God meant my surgical adventure to be my "meat tenderizer."

I discovered a spiritual illustration in my kitchen cupboard. The label of *Adolph's* Meat Tenderizer carries an extraordinary promise: "Turns commonplace cuts into gourmet products." That's exactly what I use it for.

I can transform inexpensive hamburger or economy portions of roast or steak into tasty, tender meals that pass for expensive cuts if I sprinkle them first with Meat Tenderizer.

Yes, Lord, I'm just a commonplace cut. I'd like to be a gourmet product fit for the Master's use. How can this happen? The jar label gives five simple steps that can also apply spiritually to God's dealings with me by His Holy Spirit.

1. *Moisten all surfaces.* The dealings of God in my life may produce *tears.* The hurts of life are real and painful. First, my heart needs to be moistened—*all* surfaces, *every part* of my life. *Lord, I am totally available to You. I hold nothing back.*

2. *Sprinkle Tenderizer generously.* The Holy Spirit is my Tenderizer. He is at work in my life transforming my heart of stone into a tender heart of flesh (Ezekiel 36:26,27). He liberally sprinkles God's promises on my hurting heart to encourage me and lift me up. *Yes, Lord, help me accept Your loving work in my life.*

3. *Pierce deeply with a fork at 1/2 inch intervals.* I don't welcome pain and affliction, but they have a redemptive purpose in my life. David testified to that experience in Psalm 119: 67, 71, 75: "Before I was afflicted I went astray, but now I keep Thy Word. It is good for me that I was afflicted, that I may learn Thy statutes." My tough, stubborn will needs to be broken, but God doesn't break my spirit. He loves me and wants to bring out His best in me. Sometimes trouble seems to invade every area of my life at once. *Every half-inch* of my world cries out for relief! *Nevertheless, I open even the deepest areas of my life to You, Lord.*

4. *Marinate.* God's work in my heart takes time.

Waiting is so hard! I am impatient to get out of my difficulty. I can't have instant everything, certainly not instant spiritual maturity. I need patience for recovery, for the return of my strength and for greater understanding of God's working in my life through this experience. David wrote, "This is my comfort in my affliction, that Thy word has revived me." As I wait for the rough times to pass, I must make the Word of God my delight so I can get through them. *Yes, Lord, give me patience while you marinate me!*

5. *Bake, broil, barbecue, roast or microwave immediately.* I'm passing through a heated situation in my life, but God knows what He is doing. He planned my tenderizing sequence to give me sensitivity, softhearted-ness and compassion for the sufferings of others.

I cry, "Enough already! Surely I don't need more heat!" However, my Lord must apply heat to separate imperfections from the pure gold. The fire of affliction is the refiner's fire. My oven experience is essential. When God's time is right, when I have learned the lessons He tries to teach me, He will deliver me from the oven of my affliction in His own way.

The result of this painful process? I will be a gourmet product, fit for my King! I will have a tender, sensitive, responsive heart of flesh toward my Lord. A heart that joyfully, quickly, genuinely responds to Him with *Yes, Lord, yes!*

The label on my jar of Meat Tenderizer says *100% Natural.* However, God's spiritual process is *100% Supernatural!* Man cannot duplicate it. Only the Holy Spirit can prepare my heart to please God.

Recently, I noticed that they have modified the ingredients in my jar of Meat Tenderizer. The new label reads: *No MSG.* They found Monosodium Glutamate to be harmful to our health. In God's process of maturing me through trials, the Holy Spirit is the only active ingredient—perfectly pure and always working for my good.

Yes, Lord, I trust Your loving work in my life! I'm grateful for Your divine culinary attention! With David I acknowledge, "I know, O Lord, that Thy judgments are righteous, and that in faithfulness Thou hast afflicted me." (Psalm 119:75) ◆

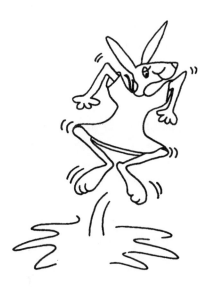

My Personal Workout

1. What "oil" do I find in my "water" that God turns into good?

2. Under what circumstances am I prone to have imaginary anxieties? How has 2 Corinthians 10:5 worked for me?

3. How have I kept my thoughts from turning inward to my problem?

4. Plan to spend some extended time quietly before the Lord to examine your life by the questions in the "Take Time Out" section in The Back of the Book. Review your answers and progress periodically.

5. What personal "a o s" can I thankfully list at this point?

6. How can I "set my house in order" in practical, financial, spiritual and relational ways?

7. If I have a Last Will, I will check it to be sure it reflects my current wishes and is valid in the State where I reside. If I don't have a Last Will, I will take immediate steps to write one.

8. What routine "w y d s" do I consider purely secular or merely time-consuming? How can I apply 1 Corinthians 10:31 to them?

9. Does humor have enough place in my daily life? How can I improve any imbalance?

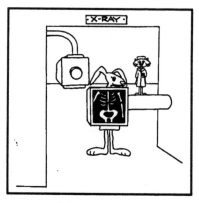

Chapter 13

Bench Warming Lessons

Why do people walk so comfortably in my former shoes, while I have to wear bedroom slippers? It surprises me when life goes right on without me! Somehow I don't want the sun to shine so brightly or people to do so well without me.

Apparently, I've seen myself as the center of my particular universe, the hub of my family's wheel, indispensable at work or in ministry. Others flattered me by reinforcing my essential image. "I don't know how we could ever get along without you. No one can take your place." Famous last words. Did I believe them? I almost threw my shoulder out of place trying to pat myself on the back.

It's a vicious circle. The more people admire me for doing so much work, the prouder I am, the harder I work and the more exhausted I become. Eventually, I lose perspective. If I'm willing to wear the self-important mask of pride, I attract more work. Worse, it weakens others who gladly step back and let me do it.

I thought the indispensable mask looked pretty good on me. It seemed to fit me well. Illness laid it aside when it laid me aside. Illness stripped a veneer from me that, in fact, had been *unbecoming.* Some of the results from its removal are unexpected fringe benefits of my illness.

The Bible tells me I shouldn't hold an exaggerated opinion of myself. Puffiness suggests ill health on both the spiritual and physical level. Being puffed up is a costly ego trip I can't afford.

> Be honest in your estimate of your-selves, measuring your value by how much faith God has given you. Just as there are many parts to our bodies, so it is with Christ's body. We are all parts of it, and it takes every one of us to make it complete, for we each have different work to do. So we belong to each other, and each needs all the others. (Romans 12:3 ᵀᴸᴮ)

Sitting on the sidelines while others star in a game which I have been playing well deflates my exaggerated self. God doesn't take away my self-esteem, just trims it down to normal size. He shows me I can't be the leading player *forever.* Everything won't fall apart if I'm not there. If others continue to depend on my performance in any aspect of life, it may stunt their emotional, mental and surely spiritual growth. Leaning on me doesn't strengthen other capable people.

I see myself now as genuinely *dispensable.* The places I occupied so importantly close easily behind me, filled by others. None of us is indispensable. We all play frail, mortal and terminal roles in life. Each of us is God's special instrument or channel. I'm unique and important to the Lord, but He can work either through me or through someone else.

Bench warming during my recovery may not be my permanent situation. As Head Coach, the Lord decides my place on His Body Team and calls me when He needs me. I must keep in good shape spiritually and be available.

I'm learning, though slowly, to act as cheer leader for every Body Team member who *is* out on the field doing a great job, perhaps even wearing *my* uniform, *my* number and *my* helmet.

Job's comforters

Sometimes I feel like talking about "it." Sometimes I don't. Sometimes I want everything to be normal, to act as if nothing out of the ordinary happened. At other times, I want to stop everybody and talk about "it."

When I want to face reality and grapple with "my big issue," I need someone to struggle through it with me. I need a sounding board, a listening ear, a sensitive heart and an encouraging word. I need God, my Ultimate Listener and Counselor, but I also need "someone with skin on," human fellowship with someone who has a fine-tuned heart. I need someone who will sense whether I want to wrestle with my problem or ignore it for the moment with normalities and trivialities.

When I'm in my normality mode, I don't need Job's comforters babbling spiritualities. I may want to play *Scrabble* or watch a TV comedy or go out to lunch. I don't want anyone to pressure me into staring my problem in the face.

Nevertheless, sometimes I do need a reminder of solid, Scriptural promises. I need someone to point me to His Bread as my only nourishment.

When I crave silence, I want to be left alone. How can I expect my friends to know what mood and what mode I'm in and relate to me according to my need? This is a complicated time for all of us! God bless the friends and family members who have developed sensitive antennae to recognize which channel I am on.

Diversion and direction

Diverting my attention from my illness is helpful at times. I wear an imaginary pair of glasses that tint my whole world with one concern—my disorder. A simple diversion by turning to ordinary routines of life is important. Life does go on, and when I can flow with its normalcy, I maintain my equilibrium.

Board games, lunch with friends, phone calls to family, nesting in an easy chair with an interesting book, (historical fiction is my favorite) sending a note of encouragement to a fellow sufferer, assembling photos in an album, baking cookies, trying a new recipe or pursuing a new or dusty hobby can have their beneficial place. Each person should find his or her workable formula for diversion. It is not mere "busy work," but part of the normal enjoyment of life.

My focus must be twofold to be healthy and productive: diversion *from* and direction *to*. I can't sweep my mind clean of thoughts about my problem. I don't live in fantasy land. I must *replace* those thoughts with other thoughts, giving them new direction. As a Christian, I must direct them upward to matters of the spirit.

In his book *Where Is God When It Hurts?* Philip Yancey quotes J. Robertson McQuilkin's reply to an elderly person questioning why God lets us become old and weak and hurting. It can apply as well to whatever weakness I experience.

> I think God has planned the strength and beauty of youth to be physical. But the strength and beauty of age [or weak bodily condition] is spiritual. We gradually lose the strength and beauty that is temporary so we'll be sure to concentrate on the strength and beauty which is forever. And so we'll be eager to leave the temporary, deteriorating part of us and be truly homesick for our eternal home. If we stayed young and strong and beautiful [and healthy], we might never want to leave.[1]
> (Brackets are the authors)

Yancey adds that to survive we must feed the spirit so it is freed beyond the body and will ultimately triumph. Despite prayers for healing, eventually every human body gives out. Jesus constantly emphasized the spirit over the body. We should see all suffering as temporary misfortune that damages only the earthly part of us. Then he quotes Alan Paton, from *CRY, The Beloved Country:*

I never thought that a Christian would be free of suffering. For our Lord suffered. I have come to believe that He suffered, not to save us from suffering, but to teach us how to bear suffering. For He knew that there is no life without suffering.[1]

I should not forget reality but nudge myself toward the reality of what is eternal and lasting beyond this life.

What do I enjoy?

Several of my friends with serious illnesses told me that they would like to have "a few more years to enjoy life." I began to wonder what it is that *I* enjoy and then to get on with doing that.

What do I enjoy? The list my friends might make is probably different from mine. With eternity's values in view I first need to sift out fleeting or useless pleasures. I really don't enjoy simple time-wasters.

Enjoying God's creation in all its aspects and enjoying human relationships would be high on *my* list. Close would be the exquisite joy of producing something creative that might last beyond my brief life. A few other "goodies" are on my list.

As I see it, the one enjoyment which will carry over into my eternal life is the answer to the catechism question, "What is the chief end [purpose] of man [humankind]?" The answer: "Man's chief end is to glorify God *and to enjoy Him forever.*" I should give that basic biblical truth my primary attention. Enjoying God is *not* a dull, religious exercise out of obligation to a distant Supreme Being. It is a warm, exciting, personal lifestyle that fulfills me, as well.

Glorifying God and enjoying Him reaches into both levels of my life: my life on earth and my eternal life. "Forever" includes both now *and* then. If this should be my important occupation right now, the transition to continuing that occupation when I leave planet Earth is no problem. I would slip from one level to the next with ease. If I have little delight and enjoyment in fellowship with God now, I'll be mighty uncomfortable spending eternity in that kind of relationship.

Busy King David, military general and leader of a nation often at war, repeatedly used the theme of "delighting" himself in the Lord in his musical poems. Apparently God was pleased because He called David a man after His own heart. *Delight* is pleasure, satisfaction, joy, happiness, fascination, enchantment, excitement—*enjoyment.* David also delighted himself in God's Word. Imagine how little of it he really had—only the first section, mostly law and history, a small part of what we call our Old Testament. I have the entire Old plus the New Testament! The two aspects of enjoyment, enjoying *God Himself* and *His Word*, should be the basis of *my* enjoyment.

Is such a relationship with God out of reach, too idealistic, or is it *priority* in my life? On what useless pursuits do I fritter away my time, letting meaningless hours and days slip through my fingers like sand? For what did God spare my life? I want to redeem my time, rein in the superfluous and target the significant in God's view. That will take discipline which I am not fully exercising yet.

O Lord, please teach me discernment at this crucial time of my life. I should be in spiritual graduate

school or holding a spiritual professorship, but I feel as
though I'm still in kindergarten. This is not the time for
me to be playing with toys!

Leaning power

A friend remarked that she would hate to be tied
down to such a restrictive routine as my scheduled
every-three-months chest x-rays. I look at it differently.
The uncertainty of my physical health keeps me on a
very short leash to my Master. He keeps me attentive to
His control.

If I walk Cindy, our German Shepherd, with a long
leash, she gets tangled around every tree and bush. She
takes her obedience to me very lightly. A short leash
keeps her close to me. She hears my quietly spoken
commands and stays under my control.

To me, close is beautiful, close is comforting.
Short accounts with God keep me leaning on Him in total
dependence. I consider it one *perk* of my weakness to be
intimately dependent on God. We highly underrate the
benefits of leaning hard on Him. People today seek to be
independent. Yet, independence from God was the
original sin, when Satan rebelled and was cast from
heaven. The desire for independence from God's instructions led to Adamic sin and disobedience. Since
then, humanity inclines toward waywardness like wandering sheep.

Left to myself without illness, pain, suffering, trials
or problems, my oceangoing vessel would get stuck on
a sand bar in shallow water.

Only when I am helpless and weak do I develop
leaning power and ability to navigate safely in deep

waters with God. Only by leaning on Jesus can I walk
uprightly. Is the Christian walk only for weaklings? Of
course, thank God! Leaning on Jesus' bosom, as the
beloved disciple John was privileged to do, is my
privilege too. "When I am weak, then am I strong" (2
Corinthians 12:10). Elisha A. Hoffman expressed it
perfectly in the words of his hymn:

> What a fellowship, what a joy divine,
> leaning on the everlasting arms;
> What a blessedness, what a peace is mine. . . .
> What have I to dread? What have I to fear? . . .
> I have blessed peace with my Lord so near. . . .
> Leaning on Jesus, leaning on Jesus,
> safe and secure from all alarms;
> Leaning, leaning, leaning on the everlasting
> arms.[2]

As a woman in labor . . .

I want to take one more look at the reality of
physical death, then I can move on to live enthusiasti-
cally anticipating the life to come. In his book cited
earlier, Philip Yancey quotes Joseph Bayly as the source
of the following analogy:

> Ironically, the one event which probably
> causes more emotional suffering than any
> other—death—is in reality a translation, a time
> for great joy when Christ's victory will be
> appropriated to each of us. Describing the
> effect of His own death, Jesus used the simile
> of a woman in labor, travailing until the mo-

ment of childbirth when all is replaced by ecstasy (John 16:21).

Each of our individual deaths can be seen as a birth. Imagine what it would be like if you had had full consciousness as a fetus and could now remember those sensations:

Your world is dark, safe, secure. You are bathed in warm liquid, cushioned from shock. You do nothing for yourself; you are fed automatically, and a murmuring heartbeat assures you that someone larger than you fills all your needs. Your life consists of simple waiting— you're not sure what to wait for, but any change seems far away and scary. You meet no sharp objects, no pain, no threatening adventures. A fine existence.

One day you feel a tug. The walls are falling in on you. Those soft cushions are now pulsing and beating against you, crushing you downwards. Your body is bent double, your limbs twisted and wrenched. You're falling, upside down. For the first time in your life, you feel pain. You're in a sea of roiling matter. There is more pressure, almost too intense to bear. Your head is squeezed flat, and you are pushed harder, harder into a dark tunnel. Oh, the pain! Noise! More pressure.

You hurt all over. You hear a groaning sound and an awful, sudden fear rushes in on you. It is happening—your world is collapsing! You're sure it's the end! You see a piercing, blinding light. Cold, rough hands pull at you. A painful slap. Waaaahhhhh!

Congratulations, *you have just been born!*

Death is like that. On this end of the birth canal, it seems fiercesome, portentous, and full of pain. Death is a scary tunnel and we are being sucked toward it by a powerful force. None of us looks forward to it. We're afraid. It's full of pressure, pain, darkness . . . the unknown. But beyond the darkness and the pain *there's a whole new world outside!* When we wake up after death in that bright new world, our tears and hurts will be mere memories. [3]

Yancey comments that though the new world is so much better than this one, we have no vocabulary to accurately describe it. The best the Bible writers can tell us is that we will be in the presence of God and see Him face to face. Our birth into new creatures will be complete.

We shall be changed (transformed). For this perishable [part of us] must put on the imperishable [nature], and this mortal [part of us]—this nature that is capable of dying—must put on immortality (freedom from death).

And when this perishable puts on the imperishable and this [that was] capable of dying puts on freedom from death, then shall be fulfilled the Scripture that says, Death is swallowed up (utterly vanquished, forever) in and unto victory.

O death, where is your victory? O death, where is your sting? . . .But thanks be to God, Who gives us the victory—making us conquer-

ors—through our Lord Jesus Christ. (1
Corinthians 15:52-55,57 ^Amplified^)

> Whatever we may have to go through
> now is less than nothing compared with the
> magnificent future God has planned for us.
> The whole creation is on tiptoe to see the
> wonderful sight of the sons of God coming into
> their own. . . . (Romans 8:18,19 ^Phillips^)

As much as I enjoy life on planet Earth, Lord, I'm
also on tiptoes of anticipation for the time when I'll be
"coming into my own" in Your presence!

Death is beautiful?

We need to view death in a balanced way. Yes, for
the Christian it is the gateway to the next phase of our
marvelous eternal life. Let's admit it, however, the
gateway itself is *not* attractive. We should not be either
maudlin or unrealistic about it.

"Death is just a normal part of life" is an explanation we often hear, which Christians sometimes buy into
without examining its *false biblical premise.* Death is *not*
natural. We were not born to die. It isn't God's cruel
design to make us suffer, nor was it in His original
blueprint for humankind. Death is not beautiful, no
matter how we sentimentalize it or use cosmetics to
mask it. Charles Stanley sought to correct our misunder-
standing in his book, *How to Handle Adversity:*

> God never intended for man to experi-
> ence the adversity and sorrow brought about

by our forefathers' sin. Death was not a part of
God's original plan for man. Death is an interruption, God's enemy as well as man's. It is the
opposite of all He desired to accomplish. Sickness and pain are certainly no friends of God.
There was no sickness in the Garden of Eden.
The ministry of Christ bears witness to this
truth. Everywhere He went He healed the sick.
God shares our disdain for disease. Sickness is
an intruder. It had no place in God's world in
the beginning; it will have no place in His world
in the end. (Revelation 21: 3-4) Death, disease, famine, earthquakes, war—these things
were not part of God's original plan. Yet they
are part of our reality. Why? Did God lose His
grip? Has He abandoned us? Is He no longer a
good God?

[On the contrary] our reality has been
fashioned by Adam's choice to sin. And sin
always results in adversity. It is God who will
wipe away every tear. It is God who will do away
with death, crying, pain, and sorrow.[4]

For now, human death still stings our bodies and
minds. Tears and anguish are associated with it. Death
is our *enemy*, not our friend. It is not "friendly fire" but the
enemy's artillery. Under the best of circumstances, it is
not pleasant. It is wretched, often painful, prolonged. It
separates loved ones, often cutting a productive life
short and seems wasteful. We are not realistic if we
sugarcoat it with sentimentalities. Sickness often associated with it is dreadful.

What is *beyond* that gateway is what we must
focus our attention and desires on. Jesus Christ con-

quered death when He took the sting upon Himself and lead the way by His own agonizing death *and resurrection.*

> "Death is swallowed up in victory. O death, where is your victory? O death, where is your sting?" The sting of death is sin, and the power of sin is the law; but *thanks be to God*, who *gives us the victory* through our Lord Jesus Christ. (1 Corinthians 15:54-57)

Worship the King

I've learned much more about worship during my illness. Does that seem strange? The alternative is to slam the door on God, complain against Him in anger, doubt and rebellion and withdraw into myself. If I seek wholeness of spirit and body, I must maintain an open door policy toward God.

No, I don't run to worship in church each time the doors open. Worship is becoming my way of life, permeating my days and pervading my nights. I never hang up the phone on God. I can be in constant, intimate touch with my Lord no matter what else I'm doing. I don't get in touch with God in the morning like winding up a mechanical toy, then letting His presence wind down as the spring slackens. My worship and celebration of God are more like an old-fashioned trolley car which keeps in unbroken contact with the power line running above it. That is abiding in Christ.

Jesus said: "Abide in Me and I in you . . . apart from Me, you can do nothing. . . . If you abide in Me, and

My words abide in you, ask whatever you wish, and it shall be done for you" (John 15:4-7).

Asking, however, isn't the greatest part of communication with God. It is more like thanking God, praising Him, worshiping, consciously appreciating God's presence, celebrating Him and affirming His work in my life. I sing to Him and about Him, not always with my vocal chords, but in my mind and in my spirit where I form the words silently. As I delight myself in the Lord, He cheers my heart no matter what my circumstances.

All my springs of joy are in you [God]. (Psalm 87:7)

And let them say continually, 'The Lord be magnified. . . .' And my tongue shall declare Thy righteousness and Thy praise all day long. (Psalm 35:27,28)

It is good to give thanks to the Lord, and to sing praises to Thy name, O Most High; to declare Thy lovingkindness in the morning and Thy faithfulness by night.
For Thou, O Lord, hast made me glad by what Thou hast done; I will sing for joy at the works of Thy hands. How great are Thy works, O Lord! Thy thoughts are very deep. (Psalm 92:4,5)

I worship God with my eyes open, walking out-of-doors, sitting quietly in thought, before falling asleep, when awakening during the night. To stay automatically tuned to the Lord's frequency keeps me from fear, worry and speculation about the future and from dwelling on my condition. He immerses me in His peace and bathes me in His comfort.

> The Lord will command His lovingkindness in the daytime; and His song will be with me in the night, a prayer to the God of my life. (Psalm 42:8)

> I will bless the Lord at all times; His praise shall continually be in my mouth. My soul shall make its boast in the Lord. . . . O taste and see that the Lord is good; How blessed is the man who takes refuge in Him! (Psalm 34:1,8)

My present worship is a rehearsal for the magnificent worship services described in The Revelation. This private experience is a delightful foretaste I can savor right now! "Holy, holy, holy is the Lord God, The Almighty. . . . Worthy art Thou, our Lord and our God, to receive glory and honor and power; for Thou didst create all things, and because of Thy will they existed, and were created" (Revelation 4:8,11).

Compassion

Jesus was "moved with compassion" in the face of human need and suffering. I'm ashamed to say, I seldom experienced that kind of feeling before my own bout with suffering. Compassion is *feeling with, identifying with* a person going through some experience. Christ could not have experienced compassion had He not "become flesh and dwelt among us," *identifying with us* "in all points."

I'm somewhat emotionally restrained by nature. I don't mean I'm detached, stoic, calloused or unfeeling toward the pain of others. I simply had never personally experienced major pain and illness. Although I'm part of Christ's body, I didn't respond as sensitively as I should have to a prick, sting or pain in another part of His body. The Lord knew it was because I missed an important class in His Life School so He gave me a chance for a makeup session.

After my own illness, I don't have to be reminded, "Remember those who are suffering, as though you were suffering as they are" (Hebrews 13:3 GNB). In the Amplified Version it reads, "since you also are liable to bodily sufferings." Compassion came with the package after I experienced illness and pain. Now I spontaneously reach out to suffering people. I don't have to whip up compassion; at times it involuntarily trickles from my eyes. My heart radiates immediately to a hurting person.

I'm thankful that I know how to be "touched with the feeling" of another's infirmities, as Christ is touched with mine. Suffering doesn't always result in the desire or ability to show compassion to others, however. One of my mature Christian friends wrote me, "I wish I could give you some words of comfort. Although I have lived in pain my entire life, I have never learned to give comfort. Sad to say, I have rarely received a genuine ministry of comfort. But I will say that on the times it has arrived, it was truly wonderful."

Instinctively, wherever there is pain, and pain will always be with us, I want to respond. I often fail at responding well, and I have much to learn. But this is a part of fulfilling the law of Christ by helping to bear another's burdens, a law or principle stemming from love not obligation.

Sometimes God intervenes for a sufferer directly, supernaturally, without the human touch, the spoken word or helping hand. More often, God chooses to use His own Christ-indwelt children as His instruments to dispense His compassionate touch and lifting power.

I have touched only the fringe of the compassion experience, but I delight in God's power flowing to me through the hem of His garment and out to others. It's exciting!

Pruning time

Recovery has become my pruning time. Not that I eat prunes every day for breakfast! God is pruning me in the way a gardener clips the shrubs, grapevines and especially fruit trees. The gardener cuts off selected branches, the unwanted extras. However, he doesn't do it because the little sprouts or new twigs are inferior or bad. On the contrary, they are especially healthy and strong. Nevertheless, if the gardener allows all the natural branches to develop because they look good, or he feels sorry to cut them off, he inhibits the strength of the main growth. The vitality of the tree or vine becomes dissipated into too many branches. When the gardener says *no* to certain shoots and *yes* to others, he shows his wisdom and skill.

Does it hurt the tree to prune it? Not in the human, emotional sense of pain. The healthy improvement that results from elective surgery to the tree is worth it. The gardener does the tree a favor by his seeming rough treatment as he breaks off its little branches. If the tree could speak, it might *not* say, "Thanks, I needed that!" when the sharp clippers nip off an apparently healthy growth. The tree might not understand the need for such pain and even shriek in foliage-language, "Ouch! What did I do to deserve that?"

Jesus illustrated the process in chapter 15 of John's Gospel. He pointed out that pruning was not meant to punish a bad vine, but intended to improve a flourishing, good vine, the already fruit-bearing vine. Pruning is done to produce *more* fruit and then *much* fruit.

Jesus applied it to our spiritual lives. He said that God, the Father, is the vinedresser, the Master Gardener. Jesus is the vine, and we are the branches. He taught that our abiding in Him and He in us was indispensable for fruit-bearing. Likewise, we, as branches, must let God deal with our wild shoots. If He does not prune them, our spiritual branches become a twisted mess of unfruitful, unruly limbs.

What are those untamed shoots which the Lord must break off? They are different in each of our lives. Some people have more wild shoots, some less. I have many such unmanageable shoots popping out all over. They may be good in themselves: good works, good ideas, good plans and goals, good gifts, even good ministries. Nevertheless, I shouldn't allow them all to remain and mature according to their own inclination.

I'm not wise enough to know which branches I should detach and which I should permit to develop. Only God knows. If I don't exercise discernment to prune my unproductive shoots myself, God has to take over and break off certain branches from me.

Painful? Yes, often. Do I resist it? Usually. Do I understand why He is doing it? Often I don't. Is it necessary? Always.

> **The Lord prunes my branches by lovingly forcing me to be quiet before Him during this surgical adventure and recovery. He slows my frantic pace and provides me with time to evaluate my life.**

God closes certain doors, removes me from normal activity and isolates me from people. He shows me that I must learn to say *no* to some things which are truly good but *not His specific plan for me*. He teaches me about the gift of discernment and how to lay aside the unproductive. He gives me the assignment of forced leisure so I can get my priorities straight. Then I can continue to do His perfect will without the jumble of wild shoots.

Lord, I would like to flourish and produce heartier fruit for You. I invite You to bring Your clippers into the garden of my recovery time and do Your divine snipping. Ouch! It hurts . . . nevertheless, go ahead and prune me.

Panic polka

I'm waiting for the results of a periodic x-ray. The news about my physical condition may not always be good—as I look at it. Of course, from God's perspective, whatever the news, *it is always good.* God's will is "good and acceptable and perfect" (Romans 12:2). I have already settled it that whatever God sees fit to bring into my life is "good" and "perfect." However, it is the "acceptable" with which I struggle.

The apostle Paul set the goal: that in everything I should commend myself as a servant of God, "in much endurance, in afflictions, in hardships, in distresses . . .

by evil (bad) report and good report. . . ." (2 Corinthians 6:4,8). Sure Paul, easy for you to say.

No, I'm wrong. *It wasn't easy for you to say.* The phrases above that I left out listed many excruciating things you went through: beatings, imprisonments, tumults, labors, punishments and more. I can't even relate to most of them.

I may not always receive a good report about my condition, about the results of my treatment, about my prognosis. I keep reminding myself that eventually every human being is terminal, since God made us of mortal material. Everything tends toward deterioration. As part of the human race I could appropriately wear a sandwich board announcing, "Perishable Goods" on one side and "Fragile" on the other. "Our outer man is decaying," I'm reminded in 2 Corinthians 5:17.

I must settle it in advance: I can expect negative news of some kind down the line—if not now, then later. My physical recovery, at best, will only be temporary even if it lasts a year, ten years or a score of years. When one part of me gets patched up, before long another part will wear out, rust out, deteriorate, need major attention or overhauling. Aging, with its decline, will catch up with me. I must be realistic.

When I do get bad news, an "evil report" of some kind, it isn't time to "lose heart" or do the panic polka. It is peace time and acceptance time. It is time for the *Prayer of Serenity:*

> God grant me the serenity to accept the
>   things I cannot change,
> courage to change the things I can,
> and wisdom to know the difference.

If I can change something or do something about a bad report, Lord, give me courage and persistence. If I can't, please give me peace to accept it. My problem comes in not always knowing the difference. For that wisdom I must count on You.

If I am in Christ, He calms me. A fruit of the Spirit is self-control. Another is peace. Jesus left us peace as a specific bequest, part of His Last Will: "Peace I leave with you; My peace I give to you; not as the world gives, do I give to you. Let not your heart be troubled, nor let it be fearful" (John 14:27).

The way Jesus worded that promise implied that the state of my heart and my emotions is *under my control.* I'm not to "let" it go into emotional cardiac arrest through fear.

When a less than favorable report comes, I am to rein in my fearful heart and not let it fly off wildly. I must tie it tightly to God's promised peace. *That rope will never break!*

Come to my party

I've thrown quite a few parties during my recovery. Sometimes the people I invite don't want to come, and someone I haven't invited always shows up.

What kind of parties are they? *Pity parties!* I don't have one every day but regularly enough to become tiresome. When I feel the urge to have such a party, most people avoid me. I have the party all alone, and that's a bummer. I sit around licking my wounds and pouting. My frown reaches down almost to my knees. A *pity party* isn't really a fun time for me or anyone else who drops by.

The joy robber, ol' Satan himself, is the only one who is eager to show up. He takes for granted he's invited because he whispered the idea in my ear in the first place. When he comes to my door, he carries an armload of presents attractively wrapped for me. That's a bribe to make me let him in, and I fall for it.

I'm quite excited until I start unwrapping them. One is a 3-D gift: depression, discouragement and disappointment. The gift in the biggest box is worry. Another is a box of miscellaneous grumbles and complaints that spill out when I open it. One odd-shaped gift is full of imaginations, impatience and "what ifs." They have a bad odor! All are tied with yellow ribbons of fear. Satan tricked me by having his most important gift delivered C.O.D. It was self-pity, all wrapped up in itself. To think he made me pay to receive it!

Chuck Swindoll said that if you cuddle and nurse self-pity when it is an infant, in a short time it will grow to be a beast, a monster, a raging, coarse brute spreading the poison of bitterness and paranoia throughout your system. He said Satan is always urging us to look inward instead of outward and upward. Self-pity is the smog that pollutes and obscures the light of the Son.

Satan is offended because I don't like his gifts. He says I should keep them anyway because at a future *pity party* probably no one else will bring me gifts. He tries to trick me with one final gift—a mirror. He urges me to take a good look at myself.

Poor me! What a low self-image I see! He agrees and comments on how ill I look, then cackles at my reaction. Perhaps I will never get well, he suggests. How neglected and forgotten by others I feel! He urges me in a whisper to pull the curtains shut and give up.

I feel so pathetic that I don't even want Satan around for company. I insist that he leave my party. (That's one command he has to obey, according to James 4:7, ". . . resist the devil and he will flee from you.") As he runs out the door, that joy robber taunts me by singing a little child's ditty: "Nobody loves me, everybody hates me, I guess I'll go eat worms!" Gloom settles over the room and Satan's stench lingers.

Another knock on the door? Oh, it's God. I forgot to invite Him to my party, but He came anyway, bringing a huge basket of fruit carefully gift wrapped in gold.

God asks me whether I will accept it. I thank Him and unwrap it to find the fruit of the Spirit. (Galatians 5:22,23) The pleasant, mellow aroma is overwhelming. As I take each fruit out and put it on the party table where I stacked Satan's gifts, Satan's presents suddenly disappear. Sunshine floods the room, and a spring fragrance floats in.

God is pleased. "I have another gift for you." He hands me a mirror. *Oh no, not another mirror!* When I look into God's mirror, I see myself as a child of God created in the image of Jesus. It's like a magic mirror where I see right past the outward appearance to the heart and see as God sees. I see nothing to pity! I'm a child of The King!

Now I realize that Satan gave me a trick mirror like the kind at carnivals and fairs that distorts everything. In Satan's mirror *I didn't see my real image.*

Some say it's bad luck to break a mirror, but that doesn't apply to Satan's! I crash it to the floor, and it shatters. Everything takes on the festive atmosphere of a real "Jesus Celebration." Spontaneously I start singing, "Praise God from whom all blessings flow."

Now who's knocking at my door? All the people who declined the invitation to my *pity party!* "May we come in? A *praise party* is the kind we *want* to join!"

Strategy against enemy warfare

I have a very personal, intimate way of dealing with the invasion of cancer. I practice it with any illness. It's not a gimmick or some magic formula, no hocus-pocus. I look upon it as an affirmation of what I've asked the Lord to do in my body.

When I'm ill, my body experiences an invasion by enemy bacteria, a virus or some kind of disease germs. Or some cells in my body have gone berserk and out-of-control. In cancer certain cells become erratic and rebel against the perfect order established by their Creator. They turn on me and became lawless. Formerly my friends, they now scowl at me like an adversary. Satan, the arch rebel and initiator of turbulence, is their commander.

Greater is God who is in me, than he (Satan) who is in the world. (1 John 4:4) Since Jesus Christ is the Lord of my life, that entitles me to call for His help to battle with those irregular forces, those scoundrel cells. He has all authority to compel them to get back in line, to march in His created order—or else. If the riffraff is stubborn and beyond rehabilitation, God may herd them into His prisoner of war camp and then send them back to the Satanic domain of their tribal chief. Or He might simply line them up in front of His angelic firing squad and blast them away.

God may choose to do this in my body in various ways. He may heal me through an instant or gradual *supernatural miracle* without outside help. Zap—gone! Or He may plan to heal through *surgical removal* by the hands of a doctor. Or order the use of *chemical warfare* like chemotherapy or medication. God may conquer my illness through radiology. Some of those methods are elements or combinations of ingredients found in God's natural world which He led man to discover and apply to the healing process. Whatever reinforcements my Sovereign God wants to muster for the campaign, He's my Commander-in-chief. I'll salute and carry out His orders.

I find it helpful to visualize God routing out this physical malevolence in my body. Not in the false New Age way of conjured-up visualization, but spiritually harnessing the imagination God gave me. I pray for the will of the Lord to be done "on earth as it is in heaven." I talk with God's Command and Control in prayer and give Him complete freedom to declare His victory on the battlefield of my body. I repeatedly submit myself to His authority, (mostly to remind myself) even lifting my face and hands to Him as a symbol of my surrender.

I find it helpful to draw deep breaths to envision the Holy Spirit, pure and clean and holy, coming in His fullness to possess my entire being. He is already and always *resident*; I want Him to be *president and preeminent* to rule over my body and its organs, especially the ones that are out-of-order.

As I exhale, it is as if I exhaust any vestige of Satan in his impurity, foulness, rebellion, infection, pollution or contamination. I thank God for His promise that if I resist Satan, he *will* flee from me. In the name of Jesus, I demand that Satan loose his control of my rebellious cells or whatever is causing the chaos and anarchy of my disease or weakness.

> I do not command God to do anything. I
> would not dare. I don't insist on any particular
> plan of action. God is supreme, and I am His
> subject.

When I walk for exercise, inhaling and exhaling
deeply to build up my damaged lung, or lie at rest
breathing evenly in rhythm, I reaffirm this input-output
process in my mind and in my spirit. I verbalize these
opposites in my thoughts, not necessarily with my lips or
voice:

"In, Holy Spirit—out, invader; in, God's wholeness—out, Satan's chaos; in, God's wellness—out, all
sickness; in, peace—out, worry; in, healthy cells—out,
infection; in, order—out, rebellion; in, trust—out, fear;
march in God's order—or leave God's property; submit
to God—resist Satan," etc.

God's Word is full of contrasts: things I should put
on and take off; receive and lay aside; leave and follow
after; accept and refuse; embrace and resist. I am
comfortable with this "thinking in my heart" because the
Bible declared that as a man thinks in his heart, so is he.
(Proverbs 23:7)

The apostle Paul clearly and specifically listed the
things we should think about in Philippians 4:8. When I
saturate my mind with His thoughts, God has freedom to
do whatever work in me He chooses.

> [Christ is] far above all rule and authority
> and power and dominion, and every name that
> is named, not only in this age, but also in the
> one to come.
> And He put all things in subjection
> under His feet, and gave Him as head over all

things to the church, which is His body, the fullness of Him who fills all in all (Ephesians 1:21-23). ◆

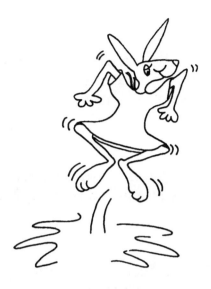

My Personal Workout

1. How have I dealt with the disappointment of not being as indispensable as I thought?

2. Do I have friends or family members who are truly sensitive to understand my mood swings and emotional needs? How have I expressed my appreciation to them? Do I make it difficult for them to care for me?

3. What diversions and enjoyments do I engage in to give balance to the more serious aspects of my recovery?

4. How has it helped me to talk about physical death and "dry run" my expectations of eternity? What questions or anxieties do I still have?

5. How have I grown in my personal experience of worship during my illness and recovery?

6. Is my degree of compassion more or less since my own experience with illness? How do I express my compassion for fellow-sufferers?

7. What has the Lord shown me that I should "prune away" in my life so I can be more spiritually productive?

8. How have I dealt with any adverse reports about my condition? How am I learning to roll such anxieties on the Lord?

9. Am I prone to have "pity parties"? What situations trigger them? How can I obtain the Lord's help to deal with self-pity?

10. Have I tried "Strategy against enemy warfare," and how has it worked for me?

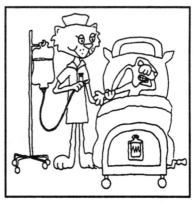

Chapter 14

Trying to Add Cubits

I try my best to do everything right during recovery: taking my medications, going for my check-ups and x-rays, forcing myself to exercise, breathing fresh air, watching my nutrition, getting enough rest and monitoring my positive outlook. I'm cooperating to the best of my ability.

As a mortal, however, I have a restricted life span and God has divinely prescribed the outer limits. We are told that every week in this country 210 men and women do reach the ripe age of 100—that's very few and still exceptional.

Formerly, most people died a lot younger (except during the Methuselah era). Now better nutrition, medical breakthroughs, surgical procedures and health habits combine to keep us on this planet longer than our ancestors. On the other hand, increased pollution, chemical food additives, drug abuse, destructive health habits, fast transportation and soft, affluent living are some negative factors pulling life expectancy downward. Heredity and accidents are contributing factors, of course.

Jesus said it realistically: "Which of you by *worrying and being anxious* can add one unit of measure [cubit] to his stature *or* to the span of his life?" (Matthew 6:27 Amplified)

Some people try to add to their bulk, stamina or speed by taking steroids, but it backfires: muscle, weight and energy may increase, but life span is cut short. Medical science can step in to prolong life to a certain extent, but life support systems, artificial body parts and transplants aren't always successful and don't last permanently.

Ultimately, for me as a Christian *the sovereignty of God* determines how long I will live. My Lord sets the timer and the wake-up alarm for heaven. I've already settled it in my heart: nothing happens to me outside His control and tender care.

> Lord, make me to know my end, and [to appreciate] the measure of my days, what it is; let me know *and* realize how frail I am—how transient is my stay here. Behold, You have made my days as [short as] handbreadths, and my lifetime is as nothing in Your sight.
>
> Truly every man at his best is merely a breath! Selah [pause, and think calmly of that]! Surely every man walks to and fro—like a shadow in a pantomime; surely for futility *and*

emptiness they are in turmoil; each one heaps up riches, not knowing who will gather them.

And now, Lord, what do I wait for *and* expect? My hope *and* expectation are in You. (Psalm 39:4-6 Amplified)

We can safely say that no one is living today who was born before 1860. They are all history—as I will be. Yes, I'll cooperate and do the best I can with who I am, what I have, who my ancestors were, where I live and what amount of time and quality of life God gives me. *Nevertheless, the cubits are not in my pocket—they are in God's!*

Not perfectly whole?

"Whole" is the King James translation of the word other versions translate "healed, completely restored, well, healthy." Dozens of references in the New Testament refer to Jesus making people "whole" of whatever illness or affliction they suffered.

"Lord Jesus, I long to be perfectly whole. . . ." the hymn writer expressed. That's the desire of my own heart and of most people who are ill. "Whole" implies complete, entire, sound and total. "Perfectly whole" and "every whit whole" is how the Bible described the unique healing results of Jesus. Not partial, fragmented or deficient.

But what if my recovery hasn't turned out to be *complete?* Suppose I'm left with weakness, partial restoration—not 100 percent? How will I manage with missing or not functioning parts? Or the prognosis that I will never be healthy from now on in this mortal body? Or that my illness may recur?

Questions bombard me. Did Jesus fail when He didn't heal me completely? Did the skill of the medical profession fall short? Was my own faith defective? Is God displeased with me? What went wrong? If Jesus can make me whole, *where's the rest of my healing?*

For a starter, I need to realize that not all healing is instantaneous or rapid whether by divine intervention or medical or surgical means. Recovery takes time. Strength returns gradually. A certain blind man saw incompletely the first time Jesus touched him. He needed a further touch by Jesus. I should be patient.

In His book *Recovery,* Chuck Swindoll writes,

> Just as hurrying the young through childhood is possible, not giving them the benefit of growing up slowly and securely, so hurrying the ill through recovery is possible, robbing them of benefits of healing slowly and permanently. [Moreover] . . . a lengthy recovery time rivets into our heads the importance of bringing our lives back from the fringes of the extreme. . . . [A prolonged period of recovery] brings a beautiful blend of insight—genuine humility, a perception of others, and an incredible sensitivity toward God.[1]

Eventually, all the people whom Jesus healed died of something, if not of another illness, ultimately from old age, accident or war. Jesus doesn't abolish the natural mortality of the human body when He heals me on a particular occasion. I've already settled in my mind that no healing or recovery is permanent, nor comes with a guarantee that I'll never be ill again either of this problem or another.

Sometimes God allows a weakness so that I may learn deeper lessons, walk with Him in greater obedience and do more quality work for Him. My weakness may be the channel to express His power through me. We know that God did not remove the apostle Paul's infirmity, whatever it was, in spite of Paul's repeated prayers. God wanted it to remain to serve His purpose.

If I experience only partial health or fractional recovery from a bodily ailment, if I'm left with residual weakness, pain, lack of vigor or recurring symptoms, I should recognize that it's part of the natural human condition. Through Christ's sufficient grace, I can accept and endure it—even joyfully.

Tim Hansel, the chronic pain survivor, wrestled with that "un-whole" condition:

> I have prayed hundreds, if not thousands, of times for the Lord to heal me—and he finally *healed me of the need to be healed.* I had discovered a peace inside the pain. I finally came to the realization that if the Lord could use this body better the way it is, then that's the way it should be. I'm quite sure I would be a different person were it not for my accident. For the past ten years, [now more than 20] I've had the opportunity to be on the steepest learning curve of my whole life. I feel like I've gotten a Ph.D. in living.[2]

I already have *spiritual wholeness* in Christ. "Ye are complete in Him" (Colossians 2:10). God will actualize my bodily wholeness when I arrive in His presence.

He will make my body "perfectly whole" without the limitations, pain and weakness of my present, corruptible mortal one. *I am whole now!* However, I lack the proper spiritual prescription lenses to see that.

I must thank God today and every day for *whatever measure* of health and freedom from pain He is giving me. It's a moment-by-moment expression of appreciation to God that transforms my attitude and keeps me from complaining.

Praise God, my cup isn't half empty—it's half full!

Is it O.K. to be *un-whole-y?*

Most people who are ill, suffering or weak hope they will recover. I say *most* because some people at least *seem* to enjoy sickness because of the attention given them or the escape from mainstream life it affords them. They are the exceptions.

My friend, who lives year after year in constant pain with times of immobility, posed her heart's question: "What if I find out I can never be physically whole and free of pain in this life? *Can God use me in my 'un-whole-y' condition?*"

The disabled, the paralyzed, those with birth defects, the physically impaired in any number of ways echo that question. They live with the probability or certainty that total or even partial recovery is not on God's agenda for them in this life.

Perhaps the question of whether or not we are *useful* to God is not the primary one. Joni Eareckson Tada suggests:

> Frankly, I think we're being redundant
> to ask God to use us. We're requesting Him to

do something He already desires to do. So maybe we should amend that prayer. Instead of praying, "Lord, use me," perhaps our prayer should be, "Lord, make me *usable*." [3]

Shouldn't our standard of measurement be, *do I please the Lord?* Perhaps we are confused about the meaning of "quality of life." People discuss that a lot these days. Should we abort a fetus because the child probably wouldn't develop the "quality of life" *we* consider acceptable? Should we do away with an aged person or allow suicide because "quality of life" has diminished? Should we allow or even help someone commit suicide because he can't stand pain or his prognosis is terminal? Should we end the life of a person of any age because they are no longer "useful" to society and their "quality of life" is substandard?

From God's perspective as revealed in the Scriptures, we can conclude that *all human life is of quality if He continues to give breath and life.* "I Am the Life" Jesus declared. Doesn't that make all life sacred, meaningful and of quality? The question of usefulness is *not for us* to measure or maneuver. It's possible to do nothing, *just to be*, and still please God. It's a matter of heart motivation and obedience. God created us, and whatever "quality of life" He grants us is His sovereign business, given in love, and not ours to decide.

Woe to the one who quarrels with his Maker—an earthenware vessel among the vessels of earth! Will the clay say to the potter, "What are you doing?" Or the thing you are making say, "He has no hands"?

Woe to him who says to a father, "What are you begetting?" Or to a woman, "To what are you giving birth?" (Isaiah 45:9,10)

Thus says the Lord, your Redeemer, and the one who formed you from the womb, "I, the Lord, am the maker of all things. . . . " (Isaiah 44:24)

For the Lord takes pleasure in His people; He will beautify the afflicted ones with salvation. (Psalm 149:4)

Even Christians are too success-oriented. We applaud accomplishment, production, proficiency and achievement. We have an attainment mindset and measure things by human standards. We conclude that health, wealth, beauty, strength, skill, talent, opportunity *and normalcy* are essential for success. God looks at it differently:

For consider your calling, brethren, that there were not many wise according to the flesh, not many mighty, not many noble;
But God has chosen the foolish things of the world to shame the wise, and God has chosen the weak things of the world to shame the things which are strong;
And the base things of the world and the despised, God has chosen, the things that are not, that He might nullify the things that are, that no man should boast before God. (1 Corinthians 1:26-29)

I don't need to thrash about complaining that I'm no use to God, that my quality of life is pathetic and I can no longer be "productive." "Just as I am, without one plea" is the way we must all come to God. Whether we are physically "un-whole-y," imperfect, limited, disabled, aged or suffer no-end-to-it affliction or pain, we can still please God and be obedient to Him. It is only when we are "unholy" that we impede His flow through us.

Whether God uses us or doesn't is entirely up to Him.

Poisonous roots

I need good nourishment during my recovery. Now that my body is rid of something which didn't belong there, or is fighting something "out-of-order," I don't want to take in anything that is not health-building. To those whose illness *was* caused by some substance abuse, the word is *nevermore!*

There's one very bitter and harmful poison that I should avoid at all costs. If I take it into my system, it's lethal. It comes from a plant or root, as most toxic substances do, but this is a *spiritual* root—none the less noxious. The writer to the Hebrews in chapter 12, verse 15 described it: "See to it that no one comes short of the grace of God; that no root of bitterness springing up causes trouble, and by it many be defiled."

Psychiatrists, medical doctors and counselors tell us that *unforgiveness* is the root of many illnesses, mental and physical, whether we are aware of it or not. I may think I have forgiven someone; I may even declare that I have. Nevertheless, if I have not *forgotten* it, caustic feelings will spring up again when least expected. The stubborn root system of bitterness grows deep and wide.

Another translation of the above verse cautions against "cultivating a root of bitterness." Is it possible that I would be so foolish as to nurture it? My time of recovery gives me an extended period on the sidelines to think, to bring up memories and to review my life.

In the leisure of my recovery period, I can either cultivate a garden or dig up a cemetery. I don't always find hidden treasure. Sometimes I unearth stinking corpses.

Because its cultivation is illegal, some growers of marijuana spend millions of dollars tunneling underground to build ultramodern, air-conditioned hothouses deep in the earth and out-of-sight. Who suspects what's underground in my life? I may have a smiling face while concealing a root of bitterness from unforgiveness, remembered hurt, offenses or injustices against me. I enshrine them in my heart. They are not dead to me, nor am I dead to them, because I kept them alive.

Am I bitter about my illness? Do I harbor hostile feelings toward others who may have contributed to it? Or against circumstances which brought it about? Or toward my heredity which determined a tendency? Am I resentful toward God? Only God knows about my hidden cache. Nevertheless, before long it will seep its putrid poison through my emotional and spiritual system. Inevitably, it will affect my physical recovery.

It will surface. Every Bible translation uses the term "spring up." I will eventually reap the destructive effects in my spiritual life and eventually in my health. My disorder will affect others, too. By it many will be defiled because it is highly contagious.

I must deal with my emotional and spiritual root system of unforgiveness before I can live in the freedom of God's perfect will for me and regain whatever measure of health He has in my future. If I don't, its poison will continue to pour into my body. "Let all bitterness and wrath and anger and clamor and slander be put away from you, along with all malice" (Ephesians 4:31).

How can I rid myself of roots that tangle and twist in the dark of my heart-earth? The Bible urges me to "walk in the light, as He Himself is in the light." (1 John 1:7) No matter how tenacious and stubborn the roots are, if I expose them to The Light of God, they will shrivel and dry. Light will terminate their life. To break the power and neutralize the bitterness of the sin of unforgiveness, I must bring it up to the light before the Lord and confess it. (1 John 1:9)

If I simply try to suppress unforgiveness by chopping off the visible part of this deadly weed, the plant soon revives. Only weed killer can slay the evil root. The blood of Christ is the guaranteed weed killer to apply to my root of bitterness. (1 John 1:7)

Why should I try any inferior alternative method or remedy?

Gray days between

During my recovery, when health is trying to push illness aside, gray days come uninvited. I call them "nothing days" because I don't seem to get anywhere. When spring tries to push winter aside, gray days often sneak between the seasons. The weather can't decide which way to go.

I'm still wading around in the dirty slush of the melting snow of my incomplete recovery. I long for the gray days to burst into sunshine.

Gray days of recovery are not my favorite days. My friend calls them "rainy days of recuperation." They make me feel moody and depressed. They are plateaus. I'd rather skip them. I'm as tired of the drag of my weakness and slow pace of recovery as I am of the bitter cold of winter, the whipping wind and drifting snow of my more acute pain. I didn't expect the recovery road to be so long. With David I cry, "O Lord, how long?" I'm impatient to hurry the season of health.

A friend described herself during recuperation as having a "go-go" brain and a "go-slow" body. Her progress fluctuated between fair days and, literally, unfair days. Sometimes her body signaled a "no-go" and refused to budge.

God, who is eternal and not subject to time, nevertheless controls the perfect timing of my situation. I want to heal quickly, to progress like a speed boat skimming along the surface of the water. But during recovery God wants me to leave surface sailing and snorkel down to the depths with the fins flapping on my feet in slow motion. There He'll show me wonders I never imagined.

I want my strength back yesterday! I don't realize that God's help and health have, in fact, been slowly dripping into my veins like the IVs in the hospital. He began the process when I first called upon Him. But shame on me—I demand express service. I want my full recovery by overnight mail or, better yet, by FAX or electronic mail. I get petulant and impatient during gray days, and my faith wears thin.

Although they come uninvited, I need those gray days of waiting to teach me endurance and perseverance, to train me to wait for God's fullness of time. Then, in the same way as the Lord draws back the curtains on His Great Drama of spring, so God will bring me back to good health or some measure of it.

Now is not the time for me to give up the struggle, to let go of the rope just because recovery time is dragging. I will encourage myself in the Lord. He never fails. He has good reasons for giving me gray days of testing and resting.

God wants me to go one step further and actually *welcome* those gray, waiting days as part of His healing process. A dark background is a most appropriate way to usher in a gorgeous spring-green scene with pink blossoms, blue skies and white clouds.

The Lord may be preparing me for something new in my life for which I need this laid back, transient, gray period to settle me down, even to equip me to help others.

Thank You, Lord, for thoughtfully providing an extended healing time. As I embrace it, may I learn to enjoy the gray days in the process.

Borrowing tomorrow

Night makes my emotions more vulnerable, especially if I can't sleep. My imagination goes into overtime. On the television screen of my mind, I see myself living tomorrow over and over. I borrow tomorrow in advance so I can "walk through it" and not be afraid when it arrives "for real." I've multiplied its terrors a hundred times. Tomorrow holds me hostage.

The strange thing about this nightmare is that I have to walk through tomorrow without God. Why? Because He *never promised* to give me strength for tomorrow *before* it arrives. "Therefore, do not be anxious for tomorrow; for tomorrow will care for itself. Each day has enough trouble of its own" (Matthew 6:34).

When it comes, but not before, God's promises *are* there for me, as is His sure presence. "As thy days, so shall thy strength be" (Deuteronomy 33:25). "My grace is sufficient for you" (2 Corinthians 12:9).

I have no business sprinting into the future by imagination to make a "dry run." The Lord's explicit promise is, "*I will go before you* and make the rough places smooth" (Isaiah 45:2).

Why do I find it so hard to live one day at a time? God gives me bite-size pieces called "days" because that's all I can chew at one time. I must savor each day slowly as prepared by God, fresh and precious. Only then am I nourished to face the future. More than one day at a time would choke me.

Some insomniacs count sheep jumping over a fence. I wonder how that idea got started. If I must count something, I'd rather count sheep *going into the safety of the fold* as my Good Shepherd guides them in with His staff. Each sheep would be one of my thoughts or concerns about tomorrow. My thoughts, like sheep, will all be safe in the protection of Jesus' fold for the night, guarded from the wolves and lions of worry or anxiety lurking in the darkness.

I don't want to be a willful or stubborn sheep jumping the fence to wander around alone and defenseless. *Lord, I'm Your restless sheep. I want to settle down in peace for the night with You because You declared, "I am The Door." When tomorrow dawns, You will be at its door with all Your strength and wisdom to help me face that day.*

Leftover limp

Most surgeries leave scars. Most of us retain some reminder even if it's only a special kind of ache whenever the weather changes. Sometimes there's an emotional reminder of the trauma or a mental flashback of our hospital adventure.

In my case, I bear a 12-inch scar, quite neatly healed because the surgeon used staples instead of stitches after surgery. I have a catch in my side whenever I sneeze or yawn from a resected rib and some diminished lung capacity. Also a shoulder ache when I drive long distances or sit too long in front of the computer. No big deal. Such discomforts are trivial.

I think of these as memory-prompters so I won't forget it really happened. More important, they serve to remind me of dealings with God, lessons I'm supposed to have learned and changes in my life perspective and direction. They are my "Jacob's limp."

Jacob, the Israeli patriarch, wrestled one night with an angel. In parting, the angel touched Jacob's thigh, and he was left with a limp for the rest of his life. It was a reminder of his dealings with God.

I tried wrestling with God for the first round of my match, but it was no contest. I happily conceded to the Lord because He has a perfect record of doing all things well for His children.

I know people who have undergone a dozen or more surgeries in their lifetime and may wonder what the fuss is all about. I'm sure they could teach me many valuable things about their hospital journeys. But they say you never forget your "first" of anything. Through this "first" for me and the recovery time following, I hope I'm developing *bigger ears* and an *enlarged heart.*

I want sensitive *ears* to hear the still, small voice of God when He speaks through my adversities. Sometimes I couldn't see meaning in my experience, but I knew God had a purpose. If I couldn't trace God's hand, I could still trust His heart. I discovered *God is not silent—* it is *I* who must learn to listen more attentively.

I want a greater *heart* of compassion for fellow-sufferers. I couldn't have bought that for any price, but I had to pay a price. When I started on my walk toward surgery, I never dreamed I would ever be thankful for such an adventure. I have now come to that point. With 20/20 hindsight, were I given the choice of going back and skipping that difficult lesson in God's classroom of life, believe it or not, I think I would still sign up for that advanced class.

Who wouldn't if their Lord was the Head Master of the school?

I'm even thankful for my "Jacob's limp," a reminder of my encounter with God.

REpeat offender?

A long list of comforting RE-words is helping me through REcovery. I'm making progress through REstoration, REfreshing, REnewing, REgaining, REpenting, REviving, REpairing, RElaxing—even REcreation. But I REsist one word and would like to REfuse it. It is the word *REpeat!*

REalistically, however, many illnesses are *REpeat*

offenders or some RElated problems. My surgeon frankly explained the strong possibility of REcurrence. It's not unusual to go through the same or similar surgery or treatment again, or REquire additional treatment. Perhaps more than once. REmission is often a temporary state.

Back to square one? I'm kept on a short leash. I circle x-ray dates at regular intervals on my calendar. I'm suspicious of symptoms that might signal the REturn of the problem. No one can guarantee full recovery from anything. We all go around in depreciating bodies. Thorns are part of the horticultural package in life and health as well as in the garden.

So, if it happens . . . ? I'll just begin the cycle again.

If God and I successfully jumped the hurdle questions at the beginning, I hope I've developed my spiritual muscles and spiritual stamina to go through it again. The same questions and struggles and the same answers apply. "Jesus Christ is the same yesterday and today, yes and forever" (Hebrews 13:8).

God offers us the same grace and strength to match any new situation. *For my good and for God's glory* is still the touchstone.

> God is *as fully in control* during the second time around—or third or fourth—as He was when I went through it the first time.

Not all race tracks are the same. On one kind of track, runners race straight ahead from starting line to finish line. No surprises, no curves. Another track is circular. The runner returns to the place where he started. In fact, the race may not be finished the first time around. He may have to run several laps around the same circle.

Still another is the marathon course where you run for the long haul through ordinary and REpetitious landscape: towns, country roads, hills, beside rivers and along highways. That's a race of endurance. The apostle Paul's words are not an understatement: "Run with endurance (patience) the race that is set before us" (Hebrews 12:1). "For you have need of endurance, so that when you have done the will of God, you may receive what was promised" (Hebrews 10:36).

Whatever kind of race track the Lord has chosen for me, my Divine Coach is cheering me on: "Run in such a way that you may win" (1 Corinthians 9:24). He was there at the Starting Line, and I know He's waiting for me at the Finish Line. He's the Alpha and Omega, the Beginning and the End. Sooner or later I'll report to Him, "I have finished the course, I have kept the faith."

Then I'll be qualified to go by the Judge's bench for my prize. "In the future there is laid up for me the crown of righteousness, which the Lord, the righteous Judge, will award to me on that day" (2 Timothy 4:7,8).

I can't lose, whatever track lies ahead in my life, if I joyfully celebrate each day of life trusting my Coach, Jesus Christ, and obediently following His instructions!

On the Ferris wheel?

Since God loves you and me so much, He will keep working on us until He has accomplished the good He wants in our lives. That's nothing short of conforming us to the image of His Son, Jesus Christ. We make the most progress toward that when we give the Lord our willing response to whatever He allows in our lives.

If we don't understand His lesson the first time, He may patiently take us through it again—and again and again. Not to be mean, but as a loving father gently instructs a child in a lesson or skill that he will need. Charles Stanley put it graphically:

> If there is something specific God wants to teach you, He will not let up until He has accomplished His will. There have been times when I felt as if I was on a Ferris wheel. Round and round I would go, experiencing the same hurt over and over again. "Lord," I would say, "what are You doing? I've already been through this." . . . . God wants to use our pain and sorrow for something positive. When we respond incorrectly, we can rest assured He will devise another way to give us a second or third chance to handle it right. [4]

Perhaps I'm a slow learner, but I'm getting one message loud and clear. What God wants is *my proper response* to things like my illness or surgical adventure: the response of a trusting child to his Father, an obedient subject to his King. I have full confidence that Jesus Christ, the Lord of my life, is in control.

Yes, Lord!

I acknowledge that I am Your property because You purchased me. "Do you not know that your body is a temple of the Holy Spirit who is in you, whom you have from God, and that you are not your own? For you have been bought with a price; therefore, glorify God in your body" (1 Corinthians 6:19).

I am also Yours because I have surrendered to You. "I urge you therefore, brethren, by the mercies of God, to present your bodies a living and holy sacrifice, acceptable to God, which is your spiritual service of worship" (Romans 12:1).

Therefore, I will accept whatever You give, Lord—with joyful heart and continued thanks. I thank You for Your goodness. "In everything give thanks; for this is God's will for you in Christ Jesus" (1 Thessalonians 5:18).

I will be content with whatever You withhold, believing it is for my good. Yes, Lord, I bow to Your loving sovereignty. "No good thing does He withhold from those who walk uprightly" (Psalm 84:11).

I will relinquish what You take whether health, companionship or material things. Yes, Lord, even those. "I have learned to be content in whatever circumstances I am. I know how to get along with humble means, and I also know how to live in prosperity; in any and every circumstance I have learned the secret . . . " (Philippians 4:11-12).

I will endure what You allow—in Your strength, not my own. Yes, Lord, without complaint. "And He said to me, 'My grace is sufficient for you, for power is perfected in weakness.' Most gladly, therefore, I will rather boast about my weaknesses, that the power of Christ may dwell in me" (2 Corinthians 12:9).

I will hold all earthly things loosely and live with eternity's values in view. Even so, come, Lord Jesus! "Since all these things are to be destroyed in this way, what sort of people ought you to be in holy conduct and godliness, looking for and hastening the coming of the day of God . . . "(2 Peter 3:11,12).

I will live today only for You, Jesus, celebrating each moment as a gift from God. Yes, Lord—to the praise of the glory of Your grace. "He died for all, that they who live should no longer live for themselves, but for Him who died and rose again on their behalf" (2 Corinthians 5:15).◆

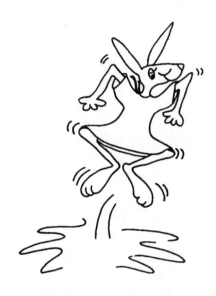

My Personal Workout

1. Do I continue to be anxious about my illness? Which of God's promises help me today?

2. What proportion of wholeness or recovery can I realistically expect? Do I thankfully accept that from the Lord?

3. Being entirely honest, how content am I with whatever quality of life God may give me?

4. Despite circumstances, am I certain of my spiritual wholeness and spiritual health?

5. Do I detect any roots of unforgiveness toward any persons or circumstances? What am I going to do about that?

6. Do I have a "leftover limp" physically or spiritually?

7. Have I learned the lessons God wanted to teach me through my illness? What were they?

8. What did I learn that might prepare me to face a recurrence of my illness or another illness?

9. What response does God want when He leads me through difficulties or allows accidents, illnesses or other adversities?

10. Am I unreservedly willing to say *Yes, Lord,* to anything He is doing in my life?

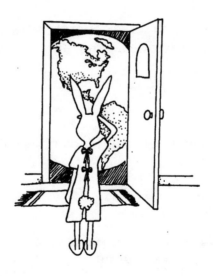

End Notes

Chapter 2

1. Stephen W. Brown, *When Your Rope Breaks*, (Nashville: Thomas Nelson Publishers, 1988), p. 63.
2. Charles Stanley, *How To Handle Adversity*, (Nashville: Thomas Nelson Publishers, 1989), pp. 187, 189-190.

Chapter 4

1. Stanley, Ibid., pp. 43, 56-57.
2. Stanley, Ibid., pp. 102-106.

Chapter 5

1. Turn to THE BACK OF THE BOOK for verses from the Bible referencing the topic of "Life After Life."
2. Turn to THE BACK OF THE BOOK for verses from the Bible referencing "Some Promises About the Future."

Chapter 8

1. Hymn: *Under His Wings,* Text: William O. Cushing, (Waco: Word Music, 1989), The Hymnal for Worship and Celebration.
2. Joni Eareckson Tada, *Glorious Intruder,* Portland: Multnomah, 1989, pp 88,90.
3. THE BACK OF THE BOOK: *"Under the Master's Command and Control."*

Chapter 9

1. Leona Choy, *Life—Stop Crowding Me!*, (Paradise: Ambassadors For Christ, Inc., 1992), p. 34.
2. Tada, Ibid., p.199.

Chapter 10

1. Stanley, Ibid., pp 187, 190.
2. Hymn: *Jesus, I am resting, resting.* Text: Jean S. Pigott, (Waco: Word Music, 1989), The Hymnal for Worship and Celebration.
3. Tim Hansel, *You Gotta Keep Dancin',* (Elgin: David C. Cook Publishing Co., 1985), p.76.
4. Henri J.M. Nouwen, *Beyond the Mirror,* (New York: The Crossroad Publishing Company, 1991), p. 69,70.
5. Robert H. Schuller, *Life's Not Fair But God is Good,* (Nashville: Thomas Nelson Publishers, 1991), pp 249-253.

Chapter 11

1. Hansel, Ibid., p. 80-81.

Chapter 12

1. Turn to THE BACK OF THE BOOK: *Take Time Out*.
2. Hymn: *He Giveth More Grace*, Text: Annie Johnson Flint, (Waco: Word Music, 1989), Hymnal for Worship and Celebration.
3. Hansel, Ibid., pp 68, 81-83.

Chapter 13

1. Philip Yancey, *Where is God When it Hurts?* (Grand Rapids: Zondervan, 1977), p. 179.
2. Hymn: *Leaning on Jesus*. Text: Elisha A. Hoffman, (Waco: Word Music, 1989), Hymnal for Worship and Celebration.
3. Yancey, Ibid., p. 180.
4. Stanley, Ibid., pp 17-18.

Chapter 14

1. Charles R. Swindoll, *Recovery: When Healing Takes Time*, (Waco: Word Books, 1985), pp 43,46.
2. Hansel, Ibid., pp 123-124.
3. Tada, Ibid., p. 234.
4. Stanley, Ibid., p. 184.

Reading Resources

Stephen W. Brown, *If God Is In Charge*, Nashville: Thomas Nelson, Inc., 1983.

Stephen W. Brown, *When Your Rope Breaks*, Nashville: Thomas Nelson, Inc., 1988.

Tim Hansel, *You Gotta Keep Dancin'*, Elgin: David C. Cook Publishing Co., 1985.

C.S. Lewis, *The Problem of Pain*, New York: Macmillan, 1940.

Edith Schaeffer, *Affliction*, Old Tappan, New Jersey: Revell, 1978.

Robert H. Schuller, *Life's Not Fair But God Is Good*, Nashville: Thomas Nelson Publishers, 1991.

Charles Stanley, *How To Handle Adversity*, Nashville: Oliver-Nelson Books, a division of Thomas Nelson, Inc. Publishers, 1989.

David Swartz, *Dancing With Broken Bones*, Colorado Springs: Navpress, 1987

Chuck Swindoll, *Recovery: When Healing Takes Time*, Waco: Word Books, 1985.

Joni Eareckson Tada, *Glorious Intruder*, Portland: Multnomah, 1989.

Philip Yancey, *Disappointment With God*, Grand Rapids: Zondervan, 1988.

Philip Yancey, *Where Is God When It Hurts?*, Grand Rapids: Zondervan, 1977.

The Back of the Book

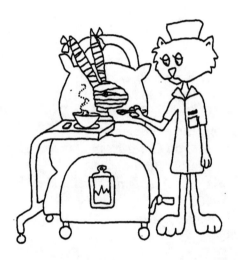

An Appendix of
Valuable Information

Life After Life

What is it? Will I have it?

This book will not make sense to you if you are not a Christian.

Unless you have a personal, life-changing faith in Jesus Christ, I can't offer you, my reader, the assurance that you will have a productive, optimistic hospital adventure or a meaningful, satisfying life.

Does that sound discouraging? It isn't! None of us can whip up enough courage or strength by self-effort or positive thinking to cope with our crises. However, in Christ we become eligible to receive God's unlimited, supernatural strength and wisdom.

Jesus Christ said of Himself that He is *the only Way, the Truth and the Life.* Does that seem too narrow? On the contrary, it's an incredibly wide, inclusive invitation. The good news is that "whosoever will may come." *Jesus offers eternal life to everyone* without any distinctions. When you receive Him, you may immediately claim every promise of God because He is now your Father. You are a born-again child of God. All of God's resources to help you live optimistically "in sickness and in health" are now available to you. You are prepared for anything life brings.

The Bible teaches that *life will never end!* That does not mean reincarnation. The simple Bible truth is that everyone will continue to live after death and spend eternity somewhere—either with Christ or without Him.

The Christian receives his personal reservation for *eternal life with Christ* the moment he accepts Christ. *He will never die* in the sense that his life will never cease. When a Christian takes his last human breath on earth, there is no interruption of his conscious life. His spirit passes immediately from life on planet Earth to life with Christ in heaven. Only the physical body dies.

Unfortunately, the person who rejects Christ, or has not yet made the personal decision to receive Him, doesn't have that bright future hope.

Don't delay making that decision. You will not have any opportunity to do so after death. However, you can receive your eternal life *right now*.

How can you do that? A religious leader once asked Jesus the same question.

> Jesus answered and said to him, 'Truly, truly, I say to you, unless one is born again, he cannot see the kingdom of God. . . .
> Whoever believes may in Him have eternal life. For God so loved the world, that He gave His only begotten Son, that whoever believes in Him should not perish, but have eternal life.
> For God did not send the Son into the world to judge the world; but that the world should be saved through Him. He who believes in Him is not judged; he who does not believe has been judged already, because he has not believed in the name of the only begotten Son of God. (Selected from the Gospel of John chapter 3)

Jesus, the Light of the world, is waiting to light up your life with His presence and power every day of your life not only in times of trouble. I invite you to consider the statements and promises from the Bible that follow and decide to accept Jesus Christ without delay, if you have not done so before. ◆

God's Road Signs to Eternal Life

"There is no distinction; for all have sinned and fall short of the glory of God" (Romans 3:22,23).

"By grace you have been saved through faith; and that not of yourselves, it is the gift of God; not as a result of works, that no one should boast" (Ephesians 2:8,9).

"Jesus answered and said to him, 'Truly, truly, I say to you, unless one is born again, he cannot see the kingdom of God' " (John 3:3).

"Behold, now is 'the acceptable time,' behold, now is 'the day of salvation' " (2 Corinthians 6:2).

"Jesus said to her, 'I am the resurrection and the life; he who believes in Me shall live even if he dies, and everyone who lives and believes in Me shall never die. Do you believe this?" (John 11:25,26).

"Therefore, if any man is in Christ, he is a new creature; the old things passed away; behold, new things have come" (2 Corinthians 5:17).

My Decision

I'm not sure of my relationship with God, and I now want to make certain. I repent of my sins and accept Jesus Christ as my personal Savior. Based on the preceding selections, I believe I am now born again and have eternal life. As a Christian, I can now, with God's help, face whatever life brings.

Name _____

Date _____

● ●

I know Jesus Christ personally. I want to affirm my belief that whatever happens in my life, my loving God has planned it for my good and for His glory.

Name _____

Date _____

Some Bible Promises About the Future for the Christian

"Jesus said, 'Let not your heart be troubled; believe in God, believe also in Me. In My Father's house are many dwelling places; if it were not so, I would have told you; for I go to prepare a place for you. And if I go and prepare a place for you, I will come again, and receive you to Myself, that where I am, there you may be also' " (John 14:1-3).

"Behold, I tell you a mystery; we shall not all sleep [die], but we shall all be changed, in a moment, in the twinkling of an eye, at the last trumpet; for the trumpet will sound, and the dead will be raised imperishable, and we shall be changed. For this perishable must put on the imperishable, and this mortal must put on immortality.

But when this perishable will have put on the imperishable, and this mortal will have put on immortality, then will come about the saying that is written, 'Death is swallowed up in victory. O death, where is your sting?' The sting of death is sin, and the power of sin is the law; but thanks be to God, who gives us the victory through our Lord Jesus Christ" (1 Corinthians 15:51-58).

"But we do not want you to be uninformed, brethren, about those who are asleep [those who died as Christians] that you may not grieve, as do the rest who have no hope. For if we believe that Jesus died and rose again, even so God will bring with Him those who have fallen asleep [died] in Jesus.

For this we say to you by the word of the Lord, that we who are alive, and remain until the coming of the Lord, shall not precede those who have fallen asleep.

For the Lord Himself will descend from heaven with a shout, with the voice of the archangel, and with the trumpet of God; and the dead in Christ shall rise first.

Then we who are alive and remain shall be caught up together with them in the clouds to meet the Lord in the air, and thus we shall always be with the Lord.

Therefore, comfort one another with these words" (1 Thessalonians 4:13-18).

"Blessed and holy is the one who has a part in the first resurrection; over these the second death has no power, but they will be priests of God and of Christ and will reign with Him for a thousand years" (Revelation 20:6).

"But the day of the Lord will come like a thief, in which the heavens will pass away with a roar and the elements will be destroyed with intense heat, and the earth and its works will be burned up. . . . But according to His promise we are looking for new heavens and a new earth, in which righteousness dwells" (2 Peter 3:10,13).

"And I saw a new heaven and a new earth; for the first heaven and the first earth passed away. . . . And He who sits on the throne said, 'Behold, I am making all things new' " (Revelation 21:1).

Under the Master's Command and Control

My Commitment: I choose You, Jesus Christ, as Lord of my life.

I put myself under Your Master Control. Reign as King of my life with full authority over my body, soul, spirit, mind, emotions and will. Rule over all that I am and all that You have given me. I accept You as Lord over every relationship, responsibility, appetite and ambition.

"I urge you, therefore, brethren, by the mercies of God, to present your bodies a living and holy sacrifice, acceptable to God, which is your spiritual service of worship" (Romans 12:1,2).

Transform Me

Continue today, Lord, to shape me into Your image through whatever circumstances You choose to bring into my life. Mold me until You finish Your chosen work in and through me.

"But we all, with unveiled face beholding as in a mirror the glory of the Lord, are being transformed into the same image from glory to glory, just as from the Lord, the Spirit" (2 Corinthians 3:18).

Live Through Me

Help me to express Your life through me as I walk in the Spirit. May I not respond in the flesh either to adversity or prosperity.

"But I say, walk by the Spirit, and you will not carry out the desire of the flesh" (Galatians 5:16).

I Want to Glorify You

I want to be a clean vessel to glorify You as I carry the treasure of Your presence and power. I want to keep myself open to the continuous filling of Your Holy Spirit. I want to bear more fruit of Your Spirit and use whatever gifts of the Spirit You give me for the building of Your kingdom.

"But we have this treasure in earthen vessels, that the surpassing greatness of the power may be of God and not from ourselves" (2 Corinthians 4:7).

Schedule for Me

Bring into my life today everything and only, whatever and whomever You will—in person, by letter, phone call, thought, impression, prayer, event or circumstance. Help me recognize that interruptions and changes are not accidental or incidental. They are my opportunities and Your appointments for my good and for Your glory.

"And we know that God causes all things to work together for good to those who love God, to those who are called according to His purpose" (Romans 8:28).

Give Me Discernment

Show me Your priorities for the hours of this day. Give me Your strength and wisdom to accomplish the tasks You've appointed specifically for me. May I be careful to abide in You and maintain my "first-love" relationship with You so that good works won't deter me from a close walk with You.

"Jesus said, 'Martha was distracted . . . worried and bothered about so many things; but only a few things are necessary, really only one' " . . . (Luke 10:40-42).

304

My Assurance

As I daily put myself under Your Master Control, I am certain that You accept my commitment. I know You will keep me on the path of Your perfect will. I am not anxious about the direction of my life nor current decisions. I trust Your love for me, the promises in Your Word, the guidance of Your Holy Spirit and Your sovereign plan for me. I am confident You are taking care of all that concerns me. I thank and praise You!

"For I am confident of this very thing, that He who began a good work in you will perfect it until the day of Christ Jesus" (Philippians 1:6). ◆

Take Time Out

A Christian's Self-evaluation

1. Do I know God's purpose for my life? Can I write it in one sentence?

2. What talents, capabilities, skills and gifts has God given me to carry out that purpose?

3. What are five of my life goals? Are they realistic? What will it take to accomplish them?

4. On a scale of 1 to 10 (10 being highest) have I been achieving my potential based on resources and opportunities God has given me?

5. Which of my unfulfilled goals remain? Are they measurable? Am I sure they are God's goals *for me* to pursue?

6. What steps could I take to accomplish my remaining life dreams and goals? Am I overlooking anything or anyone who could facilitate the accomplishment of my goals?

7. What obstacles or hindrances have I had? Are they real or imagined? Do they actually hold me back? Am I stronger by overcoming them or having to live with them?

8. What are my current limitations? Can I do anything about them? To what degree have I come to terms with any limitations? Am I willing to accept them joyfully?

9. How do I measure success? How does God measure success?

10. Do I define my self-worth in terms of my productivity or my character?

11. At what stage of life am I (early, middle, latter)? From the perspective of an average life span, how many physically, mentally, spiritually productive or alert years might lie ahead?

12. What priorities should I set in case my life is shortened?

13. What "things of the world" or "cares of this life" hinder my pursuit of eternal values and sap my time and strength? What could I eliminate or limit?

14. How efficient are my time management skills? What could I do to improve them? In what areas could I exercise more discipline?

15. What are my current responsibilities or obligations? Who gave them to me—God, others, or self-imposed? Am I giving balanced time to them—or too much or too little?

16. What cause, issue or calling grips my heart and demands my energy? Is it from God, arising from my own ambitions, or put upon me by others?

17. What specific things in my personal life or circumstances would I change if I could? Am I willing to change whatever the Lord might show me?

18. Is there anything important I feel I am presently missing in my life? Should I still go after it or accept its absence with contentment?

19. Am I passing up any specific opportunities because I lack courage or fear the cost in time, energy or money? What can I do about them?

20. Am I giving leisure, rest and wholesome enjoyment a proper place in my life? What steps can I take to achieve better balance?

21. Are most people in my life "lifter-uppers" or "down-draggers?" Do I need to make any changes in my relationships?

22. What benefits and bonus blessings has God given me in my lifetime? In the past year? Recently? Have I thanked God for them?

23. Am I more concerned about personal satisfaction and happiness, or how I can serve and encourage others?

24. What were the darkest periods of my life? Did I grow through them or did they set me back? Can I truly thank God for them?

25. What are my priority prayers? Could I be hindering God's answers in any way?

26. Is my life characterized by joy and optimism or complaint, negativism, defeat or depression?

27. How would those who know me best describe my character? How do I see myself? How do I think God sees me?

28. On a scale of 1 to 10 (10 being highest) how satisfied am I with my private spiritual life? Specifically, how can I improve my relationship with God?

29. Does any negative attitude, unforgiveness or sin come between God and me? Have I decided to deal with it?

30. Do I have a thankful, contented heart toward God, or am I frustrated about unfinished work, unfulfilled goals, broken dreams or unsatisfactory relationships?

31. Is Christ truly the center of my life, or am I focused on a cause, project, crusade, ministry, organization, person, ambition or my own desires? ◆

Just in Case . . .

Life Support Decisions

Perhaps death might not be the worst case scenario after an illness or accident. For a Christian, death is complete and immediate release from pain and the limitations of mortality. It is an anticipated, joyful continuation of eternal life with Christ in a new dimension.

A more unfortunate situation might be to linger at the point of death and to all appearances unresponsive in a coma without anyone knowing your wishes regarding life support procedures.

Newspapers, movies and magazine articles focus on stories of people lying in comas for months and years. Family members or doctors are forced to make heart-wrenching decisions, *if specific instructions and wishes were not clearly recorded in advance.*

Just in case such a situation might occur, each person should make sure to leave definite instructions. One example is on the following page. Feel free to use those suggestions or make your own corrections or additions. Be sure your lawyer approves and your statements meet the requirements of the State in which you reside.

To Whom It May Concern

Life Support Instructions

To relieve members of my family, my doctor and caregivers of responsibility or indecision concerning artificial life support, if I should become incapacitated in a clearly irreversible way, these are my instructions. I make them while I am of sound mind and body.

These instructions are to be followed if I should have a stroke, heart attack, accident, terminal illness or if advanced age or any mental or physical condition should render me incapable of making clear decisions or expressing my wishes.

If I am in a coma or unconscious and to all appearances unable to respond, I request that people nevertheless continue to treat me *as if I understood.* I request that family, friends and caregivers speak *directly to* me, not *about* me as if I was not there. In such a condition, I may hear clearly and possibly understand, although I may not be able to respond.

I wish to be told honestly, accurately and continuously about my condition.

I want someone to read Scripture to me regularly. I would like people to pray with and for me frequently. I would like to have interesting material read to me and to be kept informed about my family and people I care about. I want to know about ordinary events and current news as if I understood. Christian music may be occasionally played softly in my room. People may sing hymns in my presence.

If I am semiconscious or paralyzed and unable to speak, if I am able, I will try to nod or blink my eyes *once* to reply *yes,* and *twice* for *no,* or to squeeze a hand

312

or make a motion to indicate those answers. Anyone who addresses me should ask me questions in a way to anticipate such responses.

I request to have life support measures applied and continued *as long as there is any possibility* for at least partial recovery and/or if my pain can be relieved.

If I become brain dead or otherwise beyond hope of recovery, and God does not intervene with a miracle in answer to earnest prayer, I instruct that life support systems be stopped. Please release me in good conscience to continue my eternal life with joy in the presence of my Lord and Savior Jesus Christ.

My own additions or corrections:

_____

_____

_____

My Name: _____

Date: _____

Witness: _____

Date: _____

Witness: _____

Date: _____

Some Books by Leona Choy

Authored, edited or collaborated,
including foreign language editions

A Call To The Church From Wang Mingdao
Andrew Murray: Meet the Man Behind the Books.
   Spanish, Dutch, Chinese, Afrikaans, Korean editions
Christiana Tsai. Also Chinese edition
How to Capture and Develop Ideas for Writing
Improving Our Cross-cultural Postures:Missions on the Level
Let My People Go! Moses C.Chow with Leona Choy
No Ground. Evelyn Carter Spencer with Leona Choy
Powerlines. Also Chinese and Korean editions
Release the Poet Within! How to Launch and Improve
   Poetry Craft and Ministry
Singled Out for God's Assignment: A Widow's Valley of Learning
Touching China: Close Encounters of the Christian Kind
The Widow's Might: Strength from the ROCK
Celebrate This Moment! Prime Time is Now.
   A Trilogy of Inspirational Poetry